W0106100

Congenital Esophageal Stenosis

Ashraf Ibrahim • Talal Al-Malki

Congenital Esophageal Stenosis

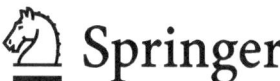 Springer

Ashraf Ibrahim
Consultant Pediatric Surgeon
Armed Forces Hospital, Southern Region
King Fahad Military Hospital
Khamis Mushait
Saudi Arabia

Talal Al-Malki
Senior Consultant Pediatric and Neonatal
Surgeon, Alhada Military Hospital
Vice President for D&Q, Taif University
Taif
Saudi Arabia

ISBN 978-3-030-10781-9   ISBN 978-3-030-10782-6   (eBook)
https://doi.org/10.1007/978-3-030-10782-6

Library of Congress Control Number: 2019935127

© Springer Nature Switzerland AG 2019
This work is subject to copyright. All rights are reserved by the Publisher, whether the whole or part of the material is concerned, specifically the rights of translation, reprinting, reuse of illustrations, recitation, broadcasting, reproduction on microfilms or in any other physical way, and transmission or information storage and retrieval, electronic adaptation, computer software, or by similar or dissimilar methodology now known or hereafter developed.
The use of general descriptive names, registered names, trademarks, service marks, etc. in this publication does not imply, even in the absence of a specific statement, that such names are exempt from the relevant protective laws and regulations and therefore free for general use.
The publisher, the authors, and the editors are safe to assume that the advice and information in this book are believed to be true and accurate at the date of publication. Neither the publisher nor the authors or the editors give a warranty, express or implied, with respect to the material contained herein or for any errors or omissions that may have been made. The publisher remains neutral with regard to jurisdictional claims in published maps and institutional affiliations.

This Springer imprint is published by the registered company Springer Nature Switzerland AG
The registered company address is: Gewerbestrasse 11, 6330 Cham, Switzerland

To my wife Aya for her love, encouragement, and support
To my daughters Hager and Sarah
To my son Ibrahim, a growing pediatric surgeon
To my grandsons Yossef and Eyad
And to my granddaughters Jasmine and Farida

A. Ibrahim

To Fatmah, our first CES patient, who taught us a lot about CES

Talal Al-Malki

Preface

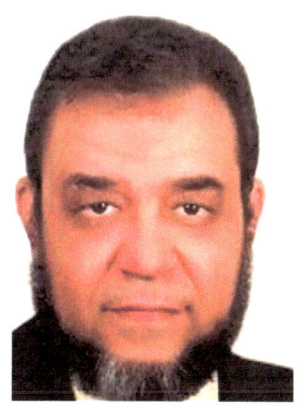

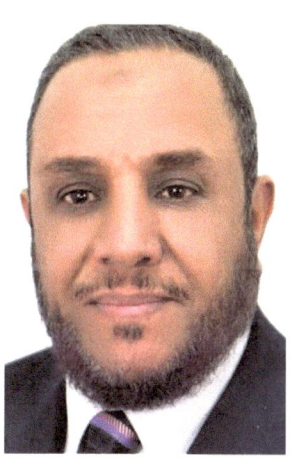

Congenital esophageal stenosis (CES) is a complex spectrum of diseases. It is our privilege to go into the depth of this topic. It is complex due to its different subtypes, different locations, and variable severity. Furthermore, almost 60% of CES are associated with esophageal atresia (EA), which adds to the complexity of the disease. The diagnosis of CES may be challenging especially in the neonates. A neonate may not pass the neonatal period without morbidities or even mortality if CES is not properly diagnosed and managed. Gastroesophageal reflux disease (GERD), dysmotility, esophageal stricture, leakage, and recurrent tracheoesophageal fistula (TEF) will add to the difficulty in managing CES. Treatment of isolated CES seems to be much easier and straightforward than that associated with EA.

Our aim is to improve the understanding of CES, its diagnosis, and management. Every effort should be made to avoid esophageal replacement surgery and to have a patient free of dysphagia. We aim at a good quality of life with the patient's own esophagus.

The aim of this comprehensive book is to help trainees and interested surgeons to develop into talented surgeons in CES management. There are enough radiographs, photographs, and tables to facilitate understanding of the topic.

To the best of our knowledge, this is the first book about CES in the literature. We hope the book will be an important addition for surgery trainees and pediatric and general surgeons.

We wish to express our deep gratitude, thankfulness, and appreciation to Professor *Nader Morad* (former chief of histopathology, College of Medicine and Medical Sciences, King Khalid University, Abha, Kingdom of Saudi Arabia), who was of great help in the histopathological part of this work.

Also, we wish to acknowledge our appreciation and gratitude to Mubarak M. Al-Shraim (Department of Pathology, College of Medicine and Medical Sciences, King Khalid University, Abha, Kingdom of Saudi Arabia) for his close supervision and valuable suggestions.

Appreciation also goes to Dr. Ahmed. *Y. Abouelyazid* (assistant professor and consultant preventive medicine, Mansoura Faculty of Medicine, Egypt) for his cooperation especially in the statistical work.

Last but not least, the authors are very thankful to Dr. Mohammed Ahmed Algathradi (consultant radiologist and pediatric radiologist at King Khalid University, Abha, Maternity and Children Hospital and Armed Forces Hospital, southern region, Saudi Arabia) for his valuable contribution in the section of external compression and vascular rings of the esophagus.

Khamis Mushait, Saudi Arabia   Ashraf Ibrahim
Taif, Saudi Arabia   Talal Al-Malki

Contents

Chapter 1
General

Introduction and Background

Congenital Esophageal Stenosis (CES) is suspected by a fixed intrinsic narrowing of the esophagus present at birth and associated with congenital malformation of the esophageal wall architecture [1]. This definition does not satisfy the whole spectrum of CES since it does not include the intra mural (membranous) nor the extramural compressions (vascular rings.. etc.). It is not necessarily symptomatic at birth. Excluding the membranous type (Membranous disease or MD) and extramural compression like vascular rings, the diagnosis of CES is only confirmed by histologic picture [2]. The histopathologic picture may show fibromuscular disease (FMD) or tracheobronchial remnants (TBR). The latter involves ciliated pseudo stratified columnar epithelium, seromucous glands or cartilage each alone or in combination [3]. There are some difficulties when talking about CES. It can be an isolated lesion or associated with other diseases mainly esophageal atresia and/or tracheoesophageal fistula (EA and/or TEF). The isolated lesion can affect any part of the esophagus proximal to the GEJ. Also, it may involve the GEJ and behaves like cardiac achalasia or peptic stricture with diagnostic challenges. The association of CES and EA and/or TEF ranges from 0.4% [1] to 14% [4–8]. The reason of this variation is due to difficulties in the diagnosis. The difficulties are due to absence of histology specimens or failure to have a high index of suspicion during the initial esophagogram. The lesion can be at the anastomotic site of EA or distal to it. FMD responds better to dilatation, whereas the TBR usually needs resection. TBR needs to be differentiated by means of histological examination at the anastomotic site or using miniprobe endoscopic ultrasonography. The extent of anastomotic CES can be very limited or it may extend down to the cardia [6]. Most of the cases reported had delayed diagnosis and management [4, 5, 9, 10]. The presentation can be early or late. Some may have a benign course whereas others may have a very stormy one that may end up with morbidity or mortality early in life [8]. Recurrent TEF and

© Springer Nature Switzerland AG 2019
A. Ibrahim, T. Al-Malki, *Congenital Esophageal Stenosis*,
https://doi.org/10.1007/978-3-030-10782-6_1

anastomotic complications after EA repair (leakage or anastomotic stricture) may be a shadow for CES due to early postoperative distal obstruction [8]. Oral feeding of the newborn can be a problem due to associated CES. Careful transanastomotic nasogastric pump feeding should be practiced until repeat esophagogram and balloon dilatation can be performed 3 weeks after primary repair. Once diagnosis is established, then to dilate or resect is a major question that needs to be answered. Dilatation is usually the initial management which may be successful and a histological diagnosis is never obtained. For all of the above mentioned reasons the true incidence of CES is difficult to assign.

Basic Notes About the Esophagus

The esophagus lies in the posterior mediastinum. It connects the pharynx to the cardia of the stomach through the esophageal hiatus of the diaphragm. It is a hollow muscular organ which propels food or fluid bolus from the pharynx to the stomach. The anatomical upper esophageal sphincter (UES) consists of cricopharyngus and the inferior pharyngeal constrictors. The lower esophageal sphincter (LES) is a specialized thickened segment of the circular muscle layer of the distal esophagus accounting for almost 90% of the basal pressure at the EGJ. Together with the crural diaphragm, it functions as an antireflux barrier [11]. During swallowing and belching, the LES relaxes briefly. This relaxation results from activation of the inhibitory innervation of the sphincter which is due to release of nitric oxide. In achalasia, there is reduction or even absence of the inhibitory innervation leading to impaired LES relaxation. In gastroesophageal reflux disease (GERD), there is failure of the antireflux barriers, with increased exposure of the esophagus to gastric acid with all of its consequences [11].

Embryology of the Esophagus and CES

The pioneer of human embryology in 1887 Wilhelm His,—cited by Kluth, in 1987 [12]—proposed that the division of the foregut is the result of the fusion of lateral ridges in the lateral wall of the foregut. The process commences in a caudal manner and ends in a cranial manner within the larynx region. This creates a septum that forms a respiratory system ventrally and a dorsal esophagus. Other researchers supported this description [13]. Later, Zaw-Tun in 1982 [14] questioned the presence of the tracheo-esophageal septum. Additionally, Kluth et al. in 1987 [12] using scanning electron microscopic techniques and microdissection did not find a septum. They posited that simple reduction of the size of the foregut triggered by a system of folds that approximates, but do not fuse causes the tracheal and esophageal development. Notably, three folds occur within the tracheoesophageal separation area including tracheoesophageal (inferior), dorsal, and laryngeal (anterocranial). The imbalance characterizing the development of the aforementioned folds would result in various types of malformation. An excessive growth of dorsal fold would account for EA and TEF. Insufficient development of the laryngeal fold would generate tracheal atresia whereas folds underdevelopment would induce full laryngo-tracheoesophageal cleft. A too close contact involving digestive and respiratory epithelia without mesoblastic interposition would lead to common wall reabsorption and isolated TEF development. Moreover, they hypothesized that late conformed esophagus ischemia would yield pure EA.

Diez-pardo et al. in 1996 [15] proved that prenatal exposure of fetal rats to Adriamycin results in tracheoesophageal spectra alongside associated malformations that are similar to those seen within humans. Possögel et al. [16] using the Adriamycin rat model, investigated the EA embryology. Their findings showed that esophagotrachea equivalent to complete tracheoesophageal cleft is the initial phase resulting in EA and TEF in their rat models. Finally the full-blown malformation is obtained through partial loss of the foregut posterior wall that tapers-off within the mediastinal mesenchyme alongside respiratory anterior wall division down towards the bronchial bifurcation level, where it constitutes the fistula and the distal esophagus. They suggested that differentiation of the tracheoesophageal separation follows an identical trend in human embryo and ordinary rat, and that tracheal bud emergence marks the septation start point and proceeds downwards. There is no generation of medial confluence of lateral ridges could be produced, and they adhered to the interpretation of tracheoesophageal separation being based on the rapid growth of the mesenchymal septum interposed between both actively elongating foregut-derived structures. The suggestion of a similar mechanism for the human and the Adriamycin-induced malformation in the view of Possögel et al. perspective is complemented; firstly, at term the animal model had a high incidence of regular EA and TEF like in human babies. Secondly, regular EA constituted the common finding, however, segregated TEF was also seen in one instance as well [15]. Thirdly, other rare forms of tracheoesophageal malformation, for instance, tracheal agenesis containing esophageal duplication and esophageal bronchi linked to EA, were observed occasionally [17]. Fourthly, Merei et al. found pure EA in 2.4% of their Adriamycin-exposed fetuses examined at term with identical anatomy as that of the sole human embryo cited with it [17]. Through the established TEF/EA model in rats, Crisera et al. discovered that distal fistula commenced as a clear equivalent tracheal anlage trifurcation [18]. They drew the conclusion that TEF grows as the tracheal trifurcation middle branch. Additionally, they posited that TEF/EA exists courtesy of a primary esophagus atresia whereas the anlage of the distal foregut is moved towards the pulmonary phenotypes in form of secondary phenomena. The latter undergoes trifurcation with its middle branch growing caudally for fistulation into the stomach.

Molecular Biology of Esophageal Atresia [19]

Embryologists concentrated on detailed description of the changes that occur in the morphology of the growing embryo. They concentrated on cell differentiation, differential cell growth, body layer folding, fusion and division. Advances in genetics and molecular biology lead to focusing on the process that occur at a cellular level and gene patterns of expression and elucidating signaling pathways. Robertson et al. in 2017 [19], highlighted some recent observations that have contributed to our understanding of the molecular biology of the embryogenesis of the foregut and its derivatives at the molecular level. They clarified that understanding the normal tracheoesophageal separation is critical to a better understanding the abnormal separation of the trachea from the esophagus that leads to EA/TEF. Previously, the most acceptable theories of the pathophysiology of EA/TEF have recently been challenged [14, 20]. Whilst those theories do not accommodate all observations, they do reflect several aspects of early tracheoesophageal separation and have served as useful models. In the mouse and rat, there is clear evidence that the bronchi develop as "lung buds" before tracheoesophageal separation occurs. This process probably driven by Fgf10 expressed in the mesenchyme overlying the tips of the primary buds. The distance between the point of tracheoesophageal separation and the pharynx is almost constant during the period of development. Accordingly, the point of separation which keeps the same distinct distance from the pharynx despite the continuous growth of the fetus and its foregut is maintained by progressive caudo-cranial apoptosis on the lateral walls of the foregut. Bmp4 expressed in the ventral mesoderm in the site which will later become the trachea and the noggin protein expressed in the dorsal endoderm of the foregut in the site which later represents the esophagus will both control the process of separation of the trachea and esophagus from each other. The dorsal endoderm may be protected from Bmp4 action by the noggin. The tracheoesophageal separation is ensured by apoptosis which seems to be critical for appropriate separation. The process of apoptosis occurs in the lateral walls at the point of tracheoesophageal separation on day 12 in the primitive foregut of the normal rat. However, it fails to occur at that time in the Adriamycin-exposed rat which is developing EA. In this model, the foregut remains a single tube showing a trachea connected to the lungs. Finally, the posterior wall of the pharynx gives origin to the upper esophageal pouch.

The Upper Esophageal Pouch

The development of the upper esophageal pouch is difficult to understand. This is due to the fact that it does not fit well with many theories of EA embryogenesis. Another reason, is that differences in its cellular properties, its innervation and intrinsic nerve supply have always been difficult to explain. The debate moreover, is further aggravated by the fact that it can elongate after birth. The first indication of the upper pouch development is indicated by apoptosis in the dorsal wall of the pharynx. The proximal esophageal pouch proliferation and extension continues until day 16 of gestation. When there is a distal TEF in humans, the proximal pouch in EA is relatively long. Also, the growth of the proximal esophageal pouch may continue during the rest of 30 weeks and after birth as well. This is also a well understood clinical observation that the proximal esophageal pouch continues to elongate significantly after birth with or without the use of bouginage [19].

Development of CES

The congenital membranous disease (MD or web or Diaphragm) has been appreciated to be an unrecognized form of EA [21]. It could be similar to membranes in other parts of the gastrointestinal tract. Histologically, the membrane is covered in both sides with squamous epithelium with an eccentric opening in most of the times.

The Fibromuscular disease or stenosis (FMD) has an unknown etiology and there is no clear embryologic or pathogenic factors to explain these lesions.

The Tracheobronchial Remnants (TBR form) occurs as part of a spectrum of anomalies, including EA/TEF, in related to tracheoesophageal separation of the foregut from the respiratory tract around the 25th embryonic day. Tracheobronchial tissue with or without cartilage is believed to become imprisoned in the wall of the esophagus and resides in the appreciated typical distal location in the esophagus due to the faster growth rate of the esophagus than the tracheobronchial tree [1]. However this is not always the case. TBR has been documented at the anastomotic site after division of the fistula and taking samples from the tip of the lower pouch (LP) [6–8]. This abnormal TBR may in times extend down into the distal pouch even down to the cardia [17].

Future Directions

New visions through the processes and the effects of gene expression as appreciated by advances in clinical genetics and molecular biology have allowed researchers tools to provide understanding of their effects on morphology. If we will have a better understanding of the normal processes, it will assist us to appreciate the mechanism and the reasons of aberrations of normal development which sometimes lead for example to EA and its related abnormalities. There is hope that at the end this knowledge will be used to prevent these anomalies [19].

Histology of the Esophagus

The esophagus consists of four layers; namely the mucosa, the submucosa, the muscularis propria and the adventia but lacks a serosal layer.

The mucosa is lined by nonkeratinized stratified squamous epithelium in all regions of the esophagus except LES, where both squamous and columnar epithelium may coexist [22]. The mucosa is the strongest layer and should be included in the anastomosis of the two pouches of the esophagus in order to have a sound anastomosis. Beneath the epithelium are the lamina propria and the longitudinally oriented muscularis mucosa. The mucus coat is separated from the submucosa by the muscularis mucosa which is the deepest layer of the mucosa. The muscularis mucosa is relatively thick especially in the lower esophagus. Its fibers are arranged longitudinally. The submucosa contains connective tissue as well as lymphocytes, plasma cells, and nerve cells (Meissner's plexus). This fine ganglionated nerve plexus is found between the sub mucosa and the circular muscle coat, called the submucous plexus of Meissner.

The submucosa contains abundant blood vessels and lymphatics. The submucosal glands are present in narrow areas near the proximal and distal ends of the esophagus. They vary in numbers from patient to patient and may be purely mucus, purely serous or mixed. They occur in three locations, at the level of the cricoids cartilage, fifth tracheal ring and at the cardiac end. The later may be simple mucus only [23]. In the regions where these glands open, the stratified squamous epithelium is replaced by columnar cells [24].

Submucosal glands are considered abnormal if they are increased in number, seromucus respiratory glands or they are found outside the submucosa [7].

The muscle coat consists of two layers, an outer longitudinal and inner circular. In the upper part of the esophagus the muscle is all striated, mixed in the middle and smooth in the lower esophagus. The circular muscle layer provides the sequential peristaltic contractions that propel food bolus towards the stomach. The ganglionated myenteric nerve plexus (plexus of Auerbach) lies between the two muscle coats. This is the more important plexus since the submucous plexus of the esophagus is sparse and consists of nerve fibers only [24].

The adventitia consists of loose connective tissue with numerous collagenous and elastic fibers at the gastroesophageal junction, which attach to the diaphragm. This is a phrenico-esophageal membrane, composed of two layers, which holds in place the fundus and the lower esophagus during diaphragmatic contractions. This membrane constitutes the only fixation of the esophagus to the diaphragmatic hiatus. The fixation is much more firm in infants than in children or adults [25, 26].

Anatomy of the Esophagus

Blood Supply of the Esophagus

The inferior thyroid artery supplies the cervical esophagus. There is an ideal submucosal plexus, which allows extensive proximal esophagus mobilization without compromising the blood supply. Notably, terminal bronchial artery branches or paired aortic esophageal arteries directly supply blood to the thoracic esophagus. It is alleged that the segmental blood supply in the lower esophageal might limit extensive lower thoracic esophagus mobilization. The intra-abdominal esophagus features an ideal supply of blood from the gastric and phrenic branches. Venous drainage occurs through the extensive sub-mucosal plexus, which carries blood from the proximal esophagus to the vena cava, and into the azygous systems from the middle esophagus. Within the distal esophagus, left gastric vein collaterals (a portal vein branch) as well as the azygos interlink within the mucosa. The connection involving the systemic venous system and the portal is important from the clinical perspective; when portal hypertension exists; variceal dilatation could occur within the region and could be the source of severe gastrointestinal hemorrhage [22].

Lymphatic Drainage

The cervical lymph nodes get drainage from the esophagus proximal third. The posterior and superior mediastinal lymph nodes get their supply from the middle third. Within the distal third, lymphatics use the left gastric arteries to move towards the gastric and celiac lymph nodes. Significant interconnections exist among the three areas [22].

Innervation of the Esophagus

The vagus nerves constitute the esophagus' motor supply. The vagal efferent fibers' cell bodies innervating the proximal striated muscles and the UES emerge within the nucleus ambiguous. The dorsal motor nucleus is the source of the fibers for the LES and distal smooth muscles. Notably, T1–T10 is the source of sympathetic sensory and motor supply towards the LES and esophagus. The vagus nerve also carries sensory innervations that feature bipolar nerves, which contain the cell bodies within the nodose ganglion projecting from there towards the brain stem [22].

Physiology of the Esophagus [22]

Propelling swallowed fluids and food into the stomach constitutes the major role of the esophagus. This is undertaken by the esophageal body's peristaltic contractions with well-timed relaxation of both the lower and upper esophageal sphincters. Other esophageal functions include clearing any refluxed components from the stomach to esophagus. Additionally, it takes part in the belching and vomiting processes.

The first deglutition stage (oral stage) is controlled voluntarily. Food undergoes chewing, combined with saliva and molded into a sized bolus that the tongue moves towards the posterior pharynx. The posterior pharynx receptors undergo activation to commence the involuntary stage. With neck and head muscle contractions, the pharyngeal constrictor muscles push the bolus to the esophagus. Concurrently, the muscles, which raise the palate and lock off and lift the larynx to avert the bolus misdirection, are activated. Immediately after the reflex activation, the UES is opened to grant passage to the bolus; afterwards, it closes quickly to block retrograde bolus passage. Notably, two main phenomena characterize the esophageal stage: The sequential contraction of the esophageal body's circular muscle that culminates in contractile waves, which move to the stomach and LES relaxation that grants passage to the bolus. The terminology–primary peristalsis is applicable to UES and LES relaxation, and related peristaltic series. Secondary peristalses constitute a peristaltic series, which exist in reaction to esophageal distensions. Its localization occurs just over the distention region. It is linked to the relaxation of the LES but not the relaxation of the UES.

The Upper Esophageal Sphincter (UES) Function

The UES acts as a barrier to pressure preventing retrograde esophageal content flow and blocking air from entering the esophagus in inspiration. Tonic UES muscle contraction forms a zone of high pressure. This is triggered by tonic neuronal discharge consisting vagal lower motor neurons. The neuronal discharge stops temporarily in deglutition to facilitate UES relaxation. This necessitates larynx anterior displacement and elevation mediated by suprahyoid muscle contractions. Relaxation takes 1 s followed by post-relaxation contraction [22].

Esophageal Body Peristalsis

Within the striated segment of the muscle, peristalsis is generated by sequentially firing vagal lower motor neurons to facilitate initial contraction of the upper segments and subsequent aboral segments. Within the segment of smooth muscles, intrinsic and extrinsic neurons can generate aboral contraction sequencing. Vagal motor fiber transection towards the esophagus involving experimental animals will eliminate peristalsis in the entire esophagus. Nevertheless, secondary peristalsis will be retained within the smooth muscles but omitted within the striated muscles. Intrinsic neuromuscular processes capable of mediating peristalsis independently, exist. When electrical stimulation is applied in vitro, smooth, circular, esophageal muscle strips indicated that the contraction latency following stimulation is brief in strips obtained from the segment of proximal smooth muscles. Latency towards contraction progressively escalates within the strips that are more distal. The contraction latency gradient is essential in the esophageal peristalsis generation. With secondary or primary peristalsis, a neutrally-based inhibition wave initially expands quickly in the esophagus. This is triggered by the nitric oxide release that generates circular smooth muscle inhibition (hyperpolarization). It is solely after recovering from the first inhibition that contraction of esophageal muscles could take place.

Therefore, the period of the first hyperpolarization could be considered crucial from the perspective of differential timing for the subsequent contractions. Notably, mechanism derangement behind the latency gradient results in dysphagia and non-peristaltic contractions [22].

Lower Esophageal Sphincter (LES) Function

The LES features a zone of high pressure caused by tonic contractions of physiologically unique circular smooth muscles at the gastro-esophageal junction (GEJ). The mean of resting LES pressure ranges from 10 to 30 mmHg above the intragastric pressure within normal adult humans. Patients having very fragile resting LES pressure are at high risk of developing gastroesophageal reflux disease (GERD). The LES resting tone emanates from myogenic factors caused by inherent muscle fiber characteristics, which cause their tonic contractions. Circulating hormones and extrinsic innervations could modify the resting tone. Esophageal distension and swallowing could trigger LES relaxation. This is influenced by vagal efferent fibers, which synapse on inhibitory myenteric plexus neurons that emit nitric oxide as the inhibitory neurotransmitter. LES relaxation takes around 5–7 s, thus allowing the bolus of food to move uninhibited from the esophagus towards the stomach. In contrast, inadequate relaxation of the LES is experienced in achalasia.

Historical Notes About CES

The first case of membranous obstruction of the upper 1/3 of the esophagus was reported by Tenon in 1791 as cited by Gupta et al. [27]. The term CES first appeared in the literature in 1826, when Rossi reported a case of distal esophageal membrane [27] Lamb was the first to describe H-type TEF with distal FMD in 1873 as cited by Margarit et al. [28]. In 1929 Abel published the first case of esophagoscopic diagnosis of a congenital membrane of the lower esophagus. CES associated with TEF was also reported by Margarit et al. [28].

The term CES then became more popular in the literature in the 1960s and early 1970s. The first case of CES due to TBR was reported in 1936 by Frey and Dusehel in a 19-year-old girl who died with the diagnosis of achalasia [29]. The first case of CES associated with an EA was reported from the Montreal Children Hospital by Dunbar in 1958 [30]. Spitz in 1973 (Fig. 1.1) was the first to demonstrate a congenital basis for distal esophageal stenosis associated with EA by showing the presence of TBR in an esophagectomy specimen [31]. This has been explained in an embryological basis. TBR is sequestrated in the esophagus during separation from the trachea at the 25th day of gestation. Normal growth of the esophagus then carried this caudally [32]. Yeung and Spitz et al. in 1992 presented eight cases of distal TBR CES. Six patients were associated with EA. They found that delayed diagnosis is a common feature. The mean lag period between presentation and definitive opera-

Fig. 1.1 Lewis Spitz was the first to demonstrate a congenital basis for the distal stenosis associated with EA by showing TBR in an esophagectomy specimen which was explained in an embryological basis

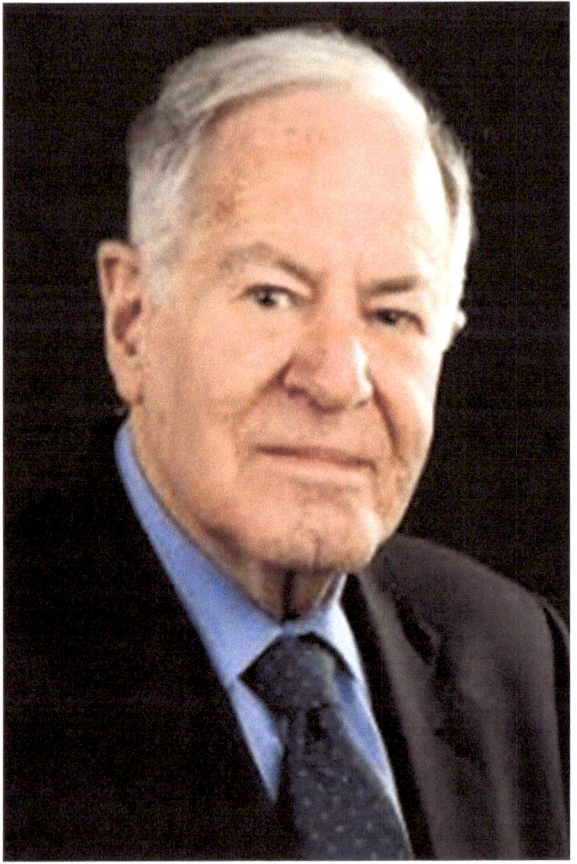

tion was 4.6 years (range 1 month to 16 years). Errors in diagnosis were common. It was an important paper to show that GERD was common in cases of distal CES and that the diagnosis was always delayed. It also concluded that TBR type of CES should be considered a possibility in patients with esophageal stricture, presumed to be inflammatory in nature, which fails to respond to standard therapy [5].

CES has been also reported in families, in father and son [33] and in sisters [34]. All had prolonged history of dysphagia and food impaction due to multiple esophageal webs.

The authors of the present study believe that those patients with prolonged history only have mild forms of CES.

References

1. Fékété CN, Backer AD, Jacob SL. Congenital esophageal stenosis, a review of 20 cases. Pediatr Surg Int. 1987;2:86–92. https://doi.org/10.1007/BF00174179.
2. Olguner M, Ozdemir T, Akgur FM, Aktuğ T. Congenital esophageal stenosis owing to tracheo-bronchial remnants: a case report. J Pediatr Surg. 1997;32:1485–7. https://doi.org/10.1016/S0022-3468(97)90570-4.

3. Hokama A, Myers NA, Kent M, Campell PE, Chow CW. Esophageal atresia with tracheo-esophageal fistula. A histopathologic study. Pediatr Surg Int. 1986;1:117–21. https://doi.org/10.1007/BF00166872.

4. Kawahara H, Imura K, Yagi M, Kubota A. Clinical characteristic of congenital oesophageal stenosis distal to associated oesophageal atresia. Surgery. 2001;129:29–3.

5. Yeung CK, Spitz L, Brereton RJ, Kiely EM, Leake J. Congenital esophageal stenosis due to tracheobronchial remnants: a rare but important association with esophageal atresia. J Pediatr Surg. 1992;27:852–5. https://doi.org/10.1016/0022-3468(92)90382-H.

6. Ibrahim AH, Al Malki TA, Hamza AF, Bahnasy AF. Congenital esophageal stenosis associated with esophageal atresia: new concepts. Pediatr Surg Int. 2007;23:533–7. https://doi.org/10.1007/00383-1927-5.

7. Al-Shraim MM, Ibrahim AHM, Al Malki TA, Morad N. Histopathologic profile of esophageal atresia and tracheoesophageal fistula. Ann Pediatr Surg. 2014;10:1–6. https://doi.org/10.1097/01.XPS.0000438124055523006.

8. Ibrahim AHM, Bazeed MF, Jamil S, Hamad HA, Abdel Raheem IM, Ashraf I. Management of congenital esophageal stenosis associated with esophageal atresia and its impact on post-operative esophageal stricture. Ann Pediatr Surg. 2016;12:36–4. https://doi.org/10.1097/01.XPS.0000482656.06000.84.

9. Teuri K, Saito T, Mitsunaga T, Nakata M, Yoshida H. Endoscopic management for congenital esophageal stenosis: a systematic review. World J Gastrointest Endosc. 2015;7(3):183–91. https://doi.org/10.4253/wige.v7.13.183.

10. Michaud L, Coutenier F, Podevin G, Bonnard A, Becmeur F, Khen-Dunlop N, et al. Characteristics and management of congenital esophageal stenosis: findings from a multi-center study. Orphanet J Rare Dis. 2013;8:186–90. https://doi.org/10.1186/1750-1172-8-186.

11. Boeckxstaens GE. The lower esophageal sphincter. Neurogastroenterol Motil. 2005;17(Suppl 1):13–21. https://doi.org/10.1111/j.1365-2982.20050066.

12. Kluth D, Steding G, Seidle W. The embryology of the foregut malformation. J Pediatr Surg. 1987;22:389–93. https://doi.org/10.1016/S0022-3468(87)80254-3.

13. Gray SW. The esophagus. In: Gray SW, Skandalakis JE, editors. Embryology for surgeons. 1st ed. Philadelphia, PA: Saunders; 1972. p. 63–99.

14. Zaw-Tun HA. The tracheoesophageal septum – fact or fantasy? Acta Anat. 1982;114:1–21.

15. Diez-Pardo JA, QiB NC, Tovar JA. A new model of experimental model of esophageal atresia and tracheoesophageal fistula: preliminary report. J Pediatr Surg. 1996;31:498–502.

16. Possögel AK, Diez-Pardo JA, Morales C, Navarro C, Tovar JA. Embryology of esophageal atresia in the Adriamycin rat model. J Pediatr Surg. 1998;33:606–12.

17. Merei J, Kotsios C, Hutson JM, Hasthorpe S. Histopathologic study of esophageal atresia and tracheoesophageal fistula in an animal model. J Pediatr Surg. 1997;32:12–4. https://doi.org/10.1016/S0022-3468(97)90081-6.

18. Crisera CA, Connelly PR, Marmureanu AR, Colen KL, Rose MI, Li M, et al. Esophageal atresia with tracheoesophageal fistula: suggested mechanism in faulty organogenesis. J Pediatr Surg. 1999;34(1):204–8. https://doi.org/10.1016/S0022-3468(99)90258-0.

19. Robertson SP, Beasley SW. The genetics and molecular biology of esophageal development. In: Till H, et al., editors. Esophageal and gastric disorders in infancy and children. Berlin: Springer; 2017. p. 9–27. https://doi.org/10.1007/978-3-642-11202-7_2.

20. Williams A, Qi BQ, Beasley SW. Three dimensional imaging clarifies the process of tracheoesophageal separation in the rat. J Pediatr Surg. 2003;38:173–7. https://doi.org/10.1053/jpsu.2003.50037.

21. Kluth D. Atlas of esophageal atresia. J Pediatr Surg. 1976;11:901–19. https://doi.org/10.1016/S0022-3468(76)80066-8.

22. Paterson WG, Mayrand S, Mercer CD. The esophagus. In: Thomson ABR, Shaffer EA, editors. First principles of gastroenterology and hepatology. Mankato, MN: CAPstone; 2012. p. 45–78.

23. Geboes K, Desmet V. Histology of the esophagus. Front Gastrointest Res. 1978;3:1. https://doi.org/10.1159/000400844.

24. Bradbury S. The digestive system. In: Hewer's text book of histology for medical students. 9th ed; 1976. p. 292.

25. Botha GSM. Mucosal folds at the cardia as a component of the gastro-esophageal junction clos-ing mechanism. Br J Surg. 1958;45(194):569–80. https://doi.org/10.1002/bjs.18004519402.
26. Bombeck CT, Dillard DH, Nyhus LM. Muscular anatomy of the gastroesophageal junction and role of phrenoesophageal ligament. Ann Surg. 1966;164(4):643–54.
27. Gupta R, Sharma P, Shukla A, Mehra S. Kluth type Iv3 membranous esophageal atresia at the middle one-third of esophagus: an extremely rare entity. J Indian Assoc Pediatr Surg. 2017;22:254–6. https://doi.org/10.4103/jiaps.JIAPS_263_16was.
28. Margarit J, Castanon M, Ribo JM, Rodo J, Muntaner A, Lee KW, et al. Congenital esophageal stenosis associated with tracheoesophageal fistula. Pediatr Surg Int. 1994;9:577–8. https://doi.org/10.1007/BF00179686.
29. Frey EK, Duschl L. Cardiospasms. Ergeb Chirur Orthop. 1936;29:637–716.
30. Dunbar JS. Congenital esophageal stenosis. Pediatr Clin N Am. 1958;5:433–55. https://doi.org/10.1016/S0031-3955(16)30660-5.
31. Spitz L. Congenital esophageal stenosis distal to associated esophageal atresia. J Pediatr Surg. 1973;8:973–4. https://doi.org/10.1016/0022-3468(91)90999-A.
32. Deiraniya AK. Congenital esophageal stenosis due to tracheobronchial remnants. Thorax. 1973;29:720–5.
33. Harrison CA, Katon RM. Familial multiple congenital esophageal rings: report of an affected father and son. Am J Gastroenterol. 1992;87:1813–5.
34. Rangel R, Lizarzabel M. Familial multiple congenital esophageal rings. Dig Dis. 1998;16:325. https://doi.org/10.1159/000016882.

Chapter 2
Histology of the Atretic Esophagus

In the literature, there is a little number of reports regarding the histology of the atretic esophagus. A study was done by Hokama et al. in 1986 [1] who examined six autopsy unoperated cases of EA and TEF as well as two surgical cases. The lower segment of the esophagus was defined as that part of the wall which is arranged into four normal layers namely adventitia, muscularis externa with myenteric plexus, submucosa, and mucosa. They defined the fistula as that portion between the tracheal connection and the transition to esophagus with normal layers. They also defined tracheobronchial elements as ciliated pseudostratified columnar epithelium, seromucus glands (in contrast to normal esophageal mucus glands) or cartilage, each alone or combined together. In the lower esophagus, Hokama et al. found a high incidence of TBR. They found TBR in five autopsy cases out of six and in the two surgical specimens. The conclusion was that TBR may be very common in EA/TEF which may lead to esophageal narrowing and dysmotility after successful surgery. This lead to the proposal that abnormal muscle coat at the fistulous end may be the cause of esophageal dysmotility. The feasibility of using the fistula in the anastomosis was questioned if this proposal is confirmed.

Merei et al. [2] from Australia, carried out a histologic study of EA and TEF in an Adriamycin animal model in 1997. All the fistulae were lined with ciliated respiratory epithelium extending to a variable distances from the origin. Occasionally, in some cases the TBR extended to as far as the stomach. Also, cartilage was sometimes seen in the wall. There was a partial or abrupt replacement of the ciliated epithelium to stratified squamous epithelium. There was absence of the muscle layer at the fistulous origin. Later, it was substituted by irregular smooth muscle fibers which were not properly arranged into normal esophageal layers. However it became regular when there was transition to normal esophageal epithelium.

Another histological study of EA/TEF in 65 cases was conducted by Dutta et al. in 2000 [3]. Thirty six cases showed that the lining epithelium was stratified squamous, pseudo stratified squamous in two and in 27 cases it was not seen. The mucous glands were seen with abnormal high number in 23 cases and showed abnormal

© Springer Nature Switzerland AG 2019
A. Ibrahim, T. Al-Malki, *Congenital Esophageal Stenosis*,
https://doi.org/10.1007/978-3-030-10782-6_2

mucin secretion (typical of respiratory glands) in 23 cases. Six cases showed dilated ducts but with increased number in four. Eight cases showed cartilage with large number of seromucus and mucous glands secreting abnormal mucin. The muscularis propria in 17 cases was poorly oriented, but well developed in 17 and in 13 was disorganized. Out of the studied cases, cartilage with mucous and seromucus glands were found in one autopsy case. While the other autopsy case, showed only mucous and seromucus glands without cartilage. There was abnormal mucin secretion in both autopsy cases. It was proposed that the TBR and disorganized muscle coat in the repaired esophagus may be part of the transition from the fistula to a normal esophagus. The TBR extent is variable and it may not be mature enough suggestion to consider this as a cause for esophageal dysmotility in each case. The authors emphasized that esophageal dysfunction may be due to presence of abnormal mucin production and abnormal numbers of glands and ducts. Esophageal stricture due to TBR which may be refractory to dilatations but responds well to resection. They presumed that these strictures are present only in the distal esophagus away from the area of anastomosis. However, this statement has been challenged. CES as we mentioned before can affect the anastomotic area [4]. Surgical specimens for histopathologic studies from the tips of the lower esophageal pouches during primary repair of EA/TEF cases could be obtained by Ibrahim et al. [4]. Histologic pictures suggestive of CES were found in ten patients out of 65 (15.4%).All of the patients did not show absent muscle layer. This excludes the possibility of using the fistula in the anastomosis. Fibromuscular disease (FMD) was seen in two cases, five had tracheobronchial remnants (TBR) without cartilage while three cases had cartilage. The epithelium was normal in seven patients and pseudostratified columnar ciliated in three cases with cartilage. These three cases showed excessive numbers of mixed respiratory glands, ducts and cartilage that extended intramurally from the submucosa to the adventitia causing significant muscle distortion (Fig. 2.1). A case with pure EA which had gastric pull up showed TBR involving the whole lower esophageal pouch reaching down to the cardia. Five patients showed mixed respira-

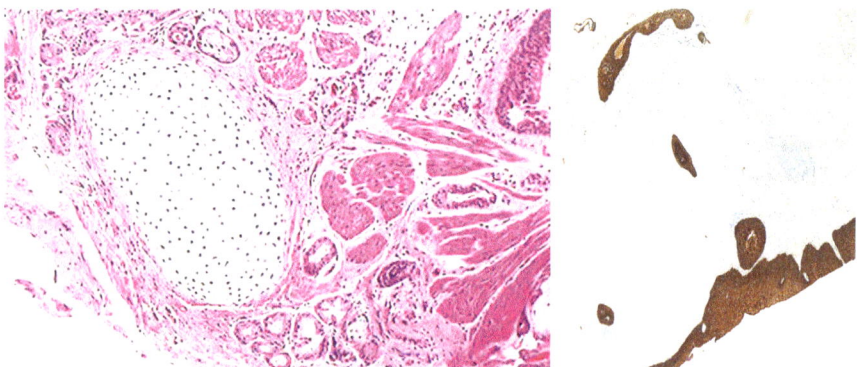

Fig. 2.1 Congenital esophageal stenosis (CES) at the anastomotic site. Samples were taken from the fistulous end of the lower esophageal pouch. The three elements of TBR namely, pseudostratified columnar ciliated epithelium, seromucus glands and cartilage are shown

tory glands without cartilage which extended from the submucosa to the adventitia causing significant muscle distortion (Fig. 2.2a, b). Seromucous or mucous glands that are increased in number and/or abnormally seated outside the submucosa were considered abnormal [4]. The other two cases were actually FMD type; were showing muscular hypertrophy and extensive fibrosis (Fig. 2.3). Tables 2.1, 2.2, and 2.3 show the details of these ten patients.

The histopathologic profile of EA and/or TEF was studied in our institution in 2014 [5]. One hundred and nineteen surgical specimens were collected from 69 consecutive cases of EA and/or TEF over a 10-year period. The results of the histology of upper and lower esophageal specimens of seven control cases are shown in Fig. 2.4a–c and Table 2.4. Those were neonates who died of major cardiac anomalies and consented for punch biopsies from the esophagus. The histopathologic profile in 69 patients with EA/TEF and two N-type TEF are shown in Table 2.5. It is important to note that only five patients had non esophageal epithelial lining. Two

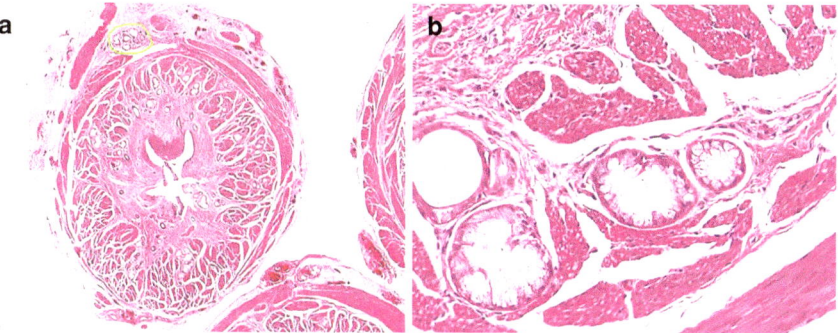

Fig. 2.2 Lower pouch photomicrograph showing (**a**) mixed respiratory glands extending outside the submucosa to the adventitia and (**b**) high power; an example of TBR without cartilage

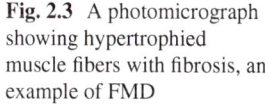

Fig. 2.3 A photomicrograph showing hypertrophied muscle fibers with fibrosis, an example of FMD

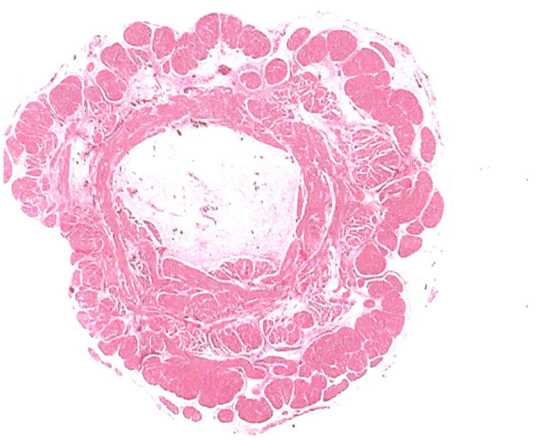

Table 2.1 GROUP I (two cases with FMD)

Criteria	Case 1: EA/TEF	Case 2: EA/TEF
Sex	Female	Female
GA/BW	33 weeks/1.9 kg	37 weeks/2.9 kg
Histopathology[a]	Unremarkable	FMD
Initial Barium	No dysmotility, GER++, No stricture	No dysmotility, GER++, no anastomotic stricture
Early post-operative period	Uneventful	Uneventful
Onset of symptoms	Three months, mainly dysphagia, aspiration and FTT	Three months, intolerance to feeds, aspiration and FTT
Subsequent Barium	• Anastomotic stricture extending distally • GER+++ • Major lower esophageal dysmotility	• Anastomotic stricture • GER+++ • Minor dysmotility
Esophagoscopy	Normal mucosa	Second degree esophagitis
Action	• Failed anti-reflux medical treatment and dilatation • Failed myotomy/Nissen fundoplication with gastrostomy at 6 months • Resection of distal stenotic area at 9 months showed FMD	• Failed medical anti-reflux measures and frequent dilatation • Nissen fundoplication at 6 months. • Esophageal diverticulectomy at 14 months • Required four dilatations
Outcome	Improved	Improved
Follow-up period	12 years	10 years

GA gestational age, *BW* birth weight, *FTT* failure to thrive

[a]Histopathology = surgical specimen from the tip of L. P at primary or delayed primary repair

had gastric epithelium alternating with esophageal epithelium (Fig. 2.5) and three with respiratory epithelium. Muscle distortion by fibrosis was more common in the upper pouch specimens than in the lower pouch (16/54 vs. 3/63 respectively). FMD with hypertrophied muscle fibers and fibrosis were seen in two upper pouch specimens and one lower pouch specimen (2.5%). TBR was seen in 11/63 lower pouch specimens (9.4%), eight without cartilage and three with cartilage.

Glands are considered abnormal if they are increased in numbers in the submucosa [3], located outside the submucosa, or they are seromucus [1, 4, 5]. Glands and/or cartilage may be seen among the muscle fibers causing distortion. They may extend well to the adventitia.

The proximal pouch mainly has striated muscle fibers and the distal has smooth muscles and no striated muscles. Transition from striated to smooth muscles is not abrupt [6]. In our study done in 2014 [5], we showed that all specimens contained muscle layers even at the fistulous end cut 3–5 mm from its origin. Only one of the two H-type fistulae was devoid of muscles. This contrasts with previous reports by Hokama [1] and Merei [2].

Table 2.2 GROUP II (five cases) TBR without cartilage

Criteria	Case 3, 4 and 5: EA/TEF	Case 6: pure EA (delayed repair at 5 mos)	Case 7: EA/TEF
Sex	Female Male Female	Female	Female
GA/BW	33 weeks/1.8 kg 37 weeks/2.4 kg 35 weeks/1.7 kg	37 weeks/2.4 kg	37 weeks/2.5 kg
Histopathology	TBR/No cartilage	TBR/No cartilage	Operated somewhere else/no pathology specimen
Initial Barium	No dysmotility in one, minor dysmotility in 2, GER++ in all, slight stricture in all	Minor dysmotility GER++ No stricture	Minor dysmotility GER++ No stricture
Early post-operative period	Uneventful	Uneventful	Uneventful
Onset of symptoms	Two months, mainly slow feeding and occasional aspiration	Ten months mainly dysphagia, FTT and recurrent aspiration	Three months, dysphagia, aspiration, FTT
Subsequent Barium	• Isolated anastomotic stricture • Minor dysmotility • GER+++	• No stricture • Minor dysmotility • GER+++	• Stricture+++ • Minor dysmotility • GER++
Esophagoscopy	Norma mucosa in all	Second degree esophagitis	Normal
Action	medical anti-reflux measures and dilatation	• Medical anti-reflux measures failed • Thal's fundoplication and temporary gastrostomy	• Failed medical anti-reflux measures • Frequent dilatations failed • Thal's/gastrostomy • Failed dilatation • Anastomotic resection → TBR without cartilage
Follow-up period/outcome	5–9 years improved	7 years improved	3 years improved

The impact of numerous mucus glands or seromucus glands without cartilage extending to the muscle layers and even to the adventitia on clinical outcome is not well understood. They may have excellent clinical outcome despite obvious radiological minor dysmotility. They respond well to medical anti reflux measures and balloon dilatation if stricture develops. Cases of cartilage present with severe stricture and/or major dysmotility requiring surgical intervention [4, 5].

Table 2.3 GROUP III. TBR with cartilage (three cases)

Criteria	Case 8: EA/TEF	Case 9: pure EA	Case 10: EA/TEF
Sex	Female	Male	Male
GA/BW	30 weeks/1.3 kg	35 weeks/2 kg	37 weeks/2.5 kg
Histopathology	TBR with cartilage	TBR with cartilage	TBR with cartilage
Initial Barium	Minor dysmotility, GER ++ Slight anastomotic stricture	–	Normal
Early post-operative period	Uneventful	–	Uneventful
Onset of symptoms	Three months, dysphagia, aspiration and FTT	–	One month/slow feeding
Subsequent Barium	• Stricture at anastomotic site extending distally • Late major dysmotility • GER ++++	–	Major esophageal dysmotility at one month No GER
Esophagoscopy	Scope could not pass	–	–
Action	• Medical anti-reflux measures and dilatations failed • Thal's fundoplication and gastrostomy at 6 mos • Recurrent symptoms • Resection of anastomotic stricture at 1 year. *Histopathology*: TBR with cartilage • Recurrent stricture • Frequent dilatations	• Failed delayed primary repair • Required resection of the whole lower esophagus and gastric pull-up • *Histopathology* of Lower. esophagus. Showed TBR with cartilage extending from the tip of L.P down to cardiac end of the esophagus	• Thal's Fundoplication • Gastrostomy at 6 weeks • Lower esophageal myectomy showed normal histology • Partial oral feeding and Gastrostomy
Follow up/ Outcome	Improved now 6 years		Improved now 4 months

Ultrastructural Changes of the Atretic Esophagus

There is scant literature data concerning the ultra-structural pathological changes within the smooth muscles in EA/TEF. Al-Shraim et al. undertook a study to show the most common ultra-structural smooth muscle cell (SMC) changes within TEF/EA [7]. Samples from the lower esophageal pouch (LEP) tip were obtained from 23 TEF/EA patients during primary repair. Each sample was divided into two parts for transmission electron microscope (TEM) and light microscope. Light microscopic investigation exhibited muscle layer distortion and significant deposition of fibrous tissue quantities in between smooth muscle fibers among 11 patients. TEM analysis

Fig. 2.4 (**a**) Control case: LEP normal mucosa and well developed muscularis mucosa. (**b**) Control case: LEP: normal mucosa and submucosa with few mucus glands. (**c**) Control case: UEP: well developed inner smooth and outer skeletal muscle

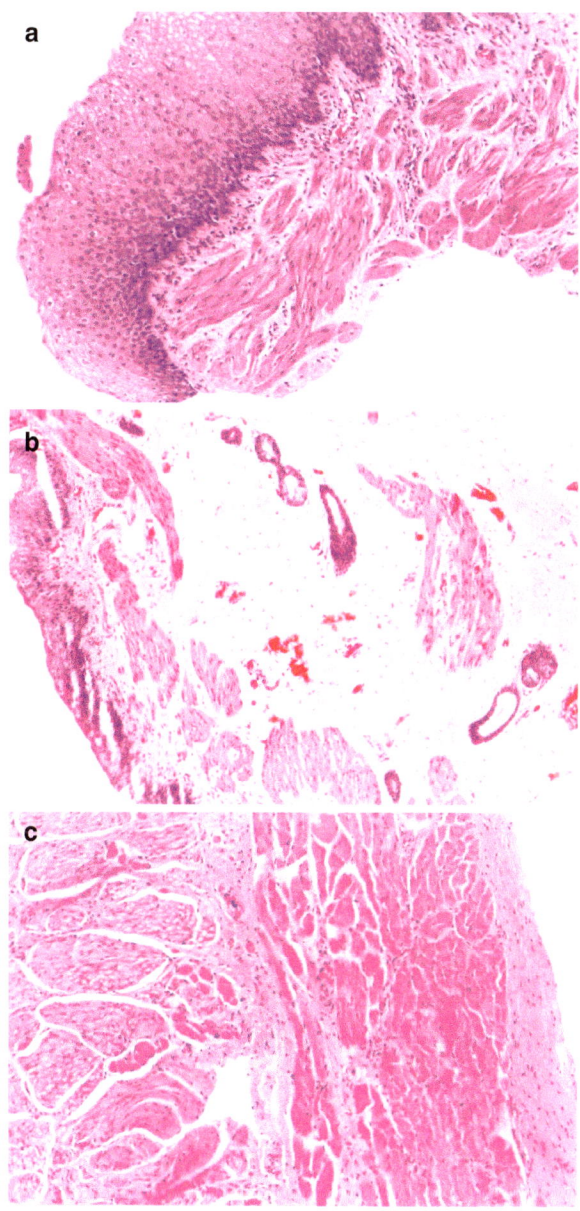

was undertaken for cases of distortion caused by fibrosis. Table 2.4 and Fig. 2.4a–c illustrate control samples under light magnification; they include well developed outer skeletal and inner smooth muscle, ordinary sub-mucosa containing small quantities of mucus glands and well-developed muscularis mucosa, and normal mucosa. Therefore, control samples exhibited normal smooth muscle arrangement and normal mucosa. The EA LEP sample exhibited fibrosis deposition distorting the

Table 2.4 histologic profile in seven control cases [5]

Histologic factor	Upper esophagus N = 7	Lower esophagus N = 7
I. Lining epithelium		
Stratified squamous	4	4
Not seen	3	3
II. Muscularis mucosa		
Thick	1	5
Thin	5	–
Not seen	1	2
III. Submucosal		
Few glands	–	2
Numerous glands	–	–
IV. Muscular layer		
Only skeletal fibers	3	–
Only smooth fibers	–	7
Inner smooth and outer skeletal	3	–
Not seen	1	–
Muscle distortion	–	–
Well-developed muscle coat	6	7
Glands/ducts	–	–
Ganglia	7	7

Table 2.5 Histologic profile in 69 patients with esophageal atresia [5]

Histologic Feature	Upper esophagus N = 54	Lower esophagus N = 63	N-Type TEF N = 2
I. Lining Epithelium			
Esophageal (Stratified Squamous)	35	43	2
Respiratory	–	3	
Gastric/Esophageal	1	1	
Not seen	18	16	
II. Muscularis Mucosa			
Well developed	22	37	
Thin	17	15	2
Not seen	15	11	
With mucous glands	2	13	2
With seromucus glands	–	2	1
III. Submucosa			
No glands or few mucus glands	43	43	
Both mucus and seromucus	–	2	1
Numerous mucous glands	9	11	2
Numerous seromucus glands	–	5	
Not seen	2	2	

Table 2.5 (continued)

Histologic Feature	Upper esophagus N = 54	Lower esophagus N = 63	N-Type TEF N = 2
IV. Muscle layers			
Absent	–	–	1
Only skeletal	7	–	
Only smooth muscle fibers	4	61	1
Inner smooth/outer skeletal	35	1	
Inner smooth/outer mixed	4	1	
Inner skeletal/outer smooth	4	–	
Well arranged muscle fibers	36	48	
Distorted muscle fibers	18	15	
Distortion by mucous glands	2	4	
Distortion by seromucus glands	–	5	
Distortion by cartilage and seromucus glands	–	3	
Distortion by fibrosis	14	2	
Hypertrophied fibers with fibrosis	2	1	
Ganglia present	54	63	–
Hypertrophied nerve trunks	–	2	–

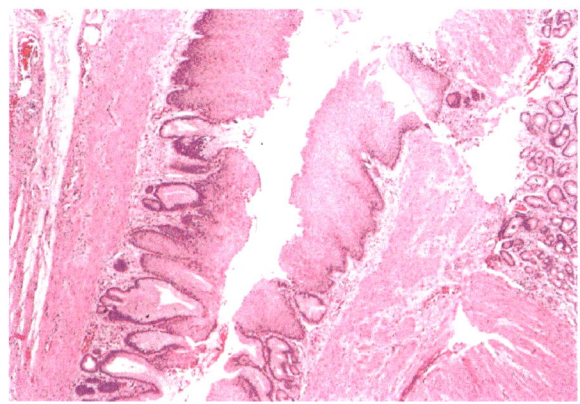

Fig. 2.5 UEP: esophageal mucosa alternating with gastric cardiac type mucosa with underlying well developed m mucosa

muscles as illustrated in Fig. 2.6. The TEM revealed within the control lower esophagus, ordinary SMC containing an intact plasmalemma with one nucleus and close contact between cells. The cytoplasm indicated regular lattice network with myosin and actin filaments. In contrast, SMCs with distortion due to fibrosis within the TEF/EA LEP revealed cell-to-cell contact loss and cytoplasm vacuolation Fig. 2.7a–d. Higher magnification showed that cytoplasmic vacuolation were due to the mitochondrial dilatation and loss of their cisternae. Some SMCs looked as either swollen with loss of lattice-like network, having lipid droplets, and small sized-vacuoles or degenerated with cytoplasmic vacuolation and formation of myelin figures.

Fig. 2.6 Representative micrographs for the histology of control and EA/TEF specimens. (**a**) A Control specimen from a normal lower esophagus showing attenuated non-keratinized stratified squamous epithelium (E) and normal arrangement of smooth muscle fibers (SM). HE stain (**b**) A specimen from EA/TEF showing distortion of smooth muscle layer (SM) and deposition of considerable amount of fibrous tissue (CT). HE stain (**c**) A specimen from EA/TEF showing smooth muscle (SM) disarrangement (yellow) and deposition of collagen fibers (red), Van Gieson's stain

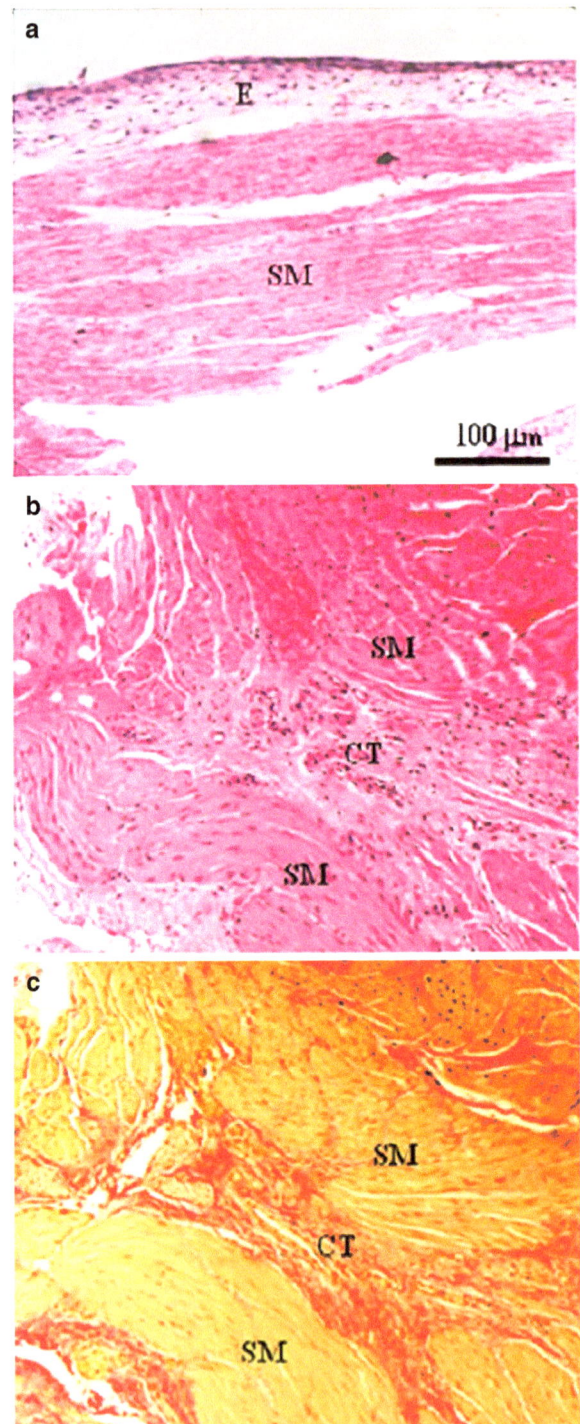

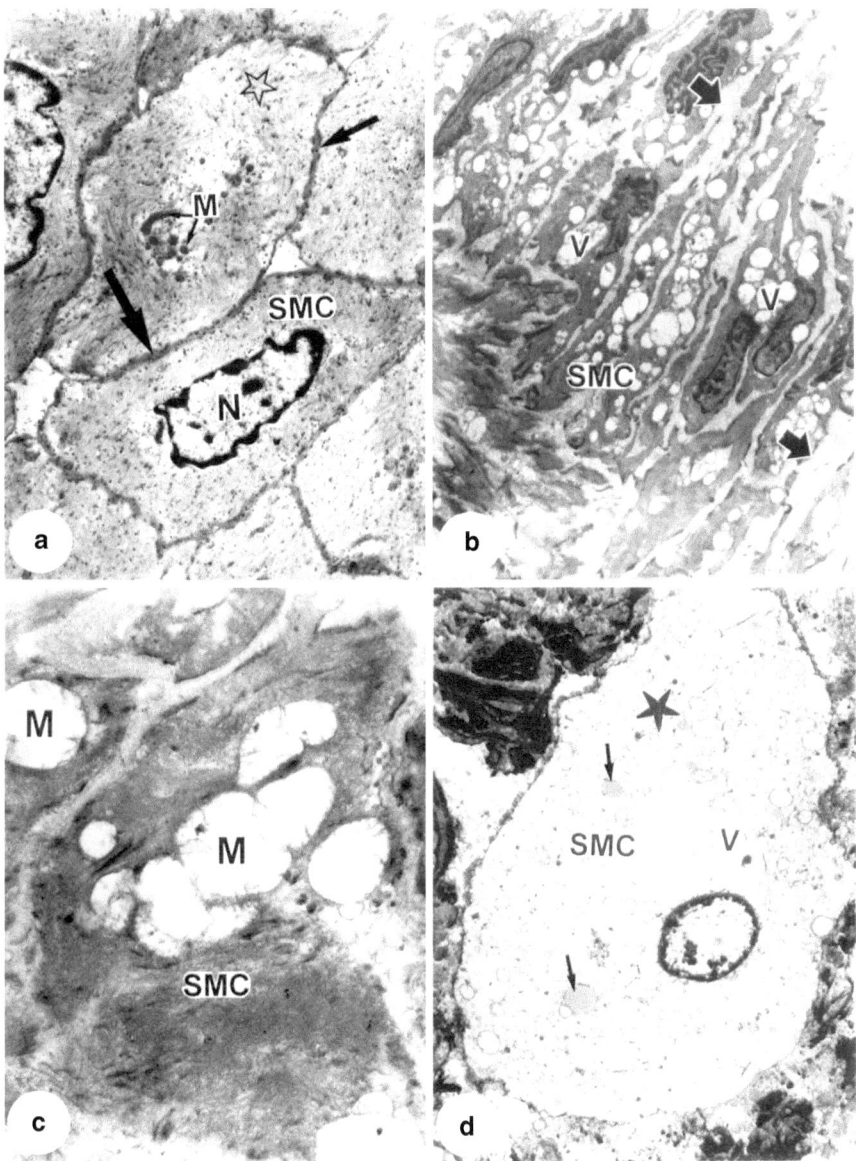

Fig. 2.7 Representative ultrastructural micrographs for SMCs in a normal lower esophagus and a LEP of EA/TEF. (**a**) Normal SMCs enclosed by an intact plasmalemma (arrow) with a single nucleus (N), few mitochondria (M), and lattice-like networks of actin and myosin filaments (stars) (magnification 9375×). (**b**) SMCs showing vacuolation (V), dysmorphic nuclei (asterisks) and loss of cell–cell contact (arrow) (magnification 6000×). (**c**) A SMC showing mitochondrial dilatation (M) and loss of mitochondrial cisternae (head arrows) (magnification 13,818×). (**d**) A swollen SMC showing loss of the lattice-like network (star), few lipid droplets (arrows), and small sized vacuoles (V). There are very fine fragments of actin and myosin (small asterisks) (magnification 4250×)

Moreover, SMCs within the TEF/EA LEP revealed formation of bulbous cytoplasmic pseudopodia processes, which connect with the body of the cell through narrow stalks. Such protrusions enlarged progressively and were detached completely from the surface of the cell as electrolucent and structureless membrane-bound bodies; this is illustrated in Fig. 2.8a–d. Some SMCs exhibited apoptotic cell death features including apoptotic body formation and nuclear condensation. The appearance of apoptotic bodies' resembled cell-membrane bound structures with nuclear fragments and cytoplasmic elements. Notably, SMCs were seen engulfing neighboring collagen fibers. Initially, SMCs extended pseudopodia projections around fibers of collagen, surrounded collagen fibers to the cytoplasm and caused their degradation in autophagic vacuoles as illustrated in Fig. 2.9a–d. It could be concluded that SMCs degeneration coupled with deposition of significant quantities of multi-cellular collagen fibers are common pathological changes within the TEF/EA LEP. Such changes might contribute towards the esophageal dysmotility pathogenesis in TEF/EA survivors.

Li et al. [8] investigated the intrinsic innervations in the fistula of patients with EA/TEF with TEM and immunohistochemistry. They discovered abnormal intrinsic dysplasia of myenteric nerve plexus coupled with an imbalanced release of neurotransmitters particularly escalated inhibitory neuropeptides expression such as vasoactive intestinal polypeptides and nitric oxide.

The interstitial cells of Cajal (ICC) constitute the essential pacemaker causing peristalsis of the intestine. They are abnormal in congenital diseases with abnormal peristalsis like gastroschisis [9], hypertrophic pyloric stenosis [10], neuronal intestinal dysplasia [11], Hirschsprung's disease [12], and pseudointestinal obstruction [13, 14].

Investigation of the ICC was undertaken in TEF/EA patients with TEM and immunohistochemistry [15]. Control samples were collected from ten patients who succumbed to non-esophageal diseases. Samples were collected from the distal and upper esophagus. Moreover, 15 full-term neonates were subjected to TEF/EA repair. Samples were obtained from distal and proximal control esophagi, the EA fistulae cases and from the upper pouch. Processing of the samples was undertaken for transmission electron microscopy, ICC identification, c-kit immunohistochemistry, hematoxylin and eosin evaluation of the c-kit positive cell frequency in 20 fields was conducted per slide with a visual score namely very high, high, medium, low, very low, and absent. Additionally, statistical analysis and morphometry were undertaken. Results indicated a very high frequency for ICC within the proximal normal esophagus in 3 scenarios, 5 indicated high and 2 indicated medium; from a distal perspective, 4 indicated high and 6 indicated medium. Within the TEF/EA upper pouch, 2 indicated high whereas 13 showed medium; within the fistula, 1 indicated nil, 3 indicated very low, 6 indicated low, and 5 indicated medium. The aforementioned results were confirmed through morphometry. Comparison between fistula and upper pouch against lower and proximal esophagus indicated variations that were statistically significant. Furthermore, TEM revealed ICC immaturity within TEF/EA. Overall, it

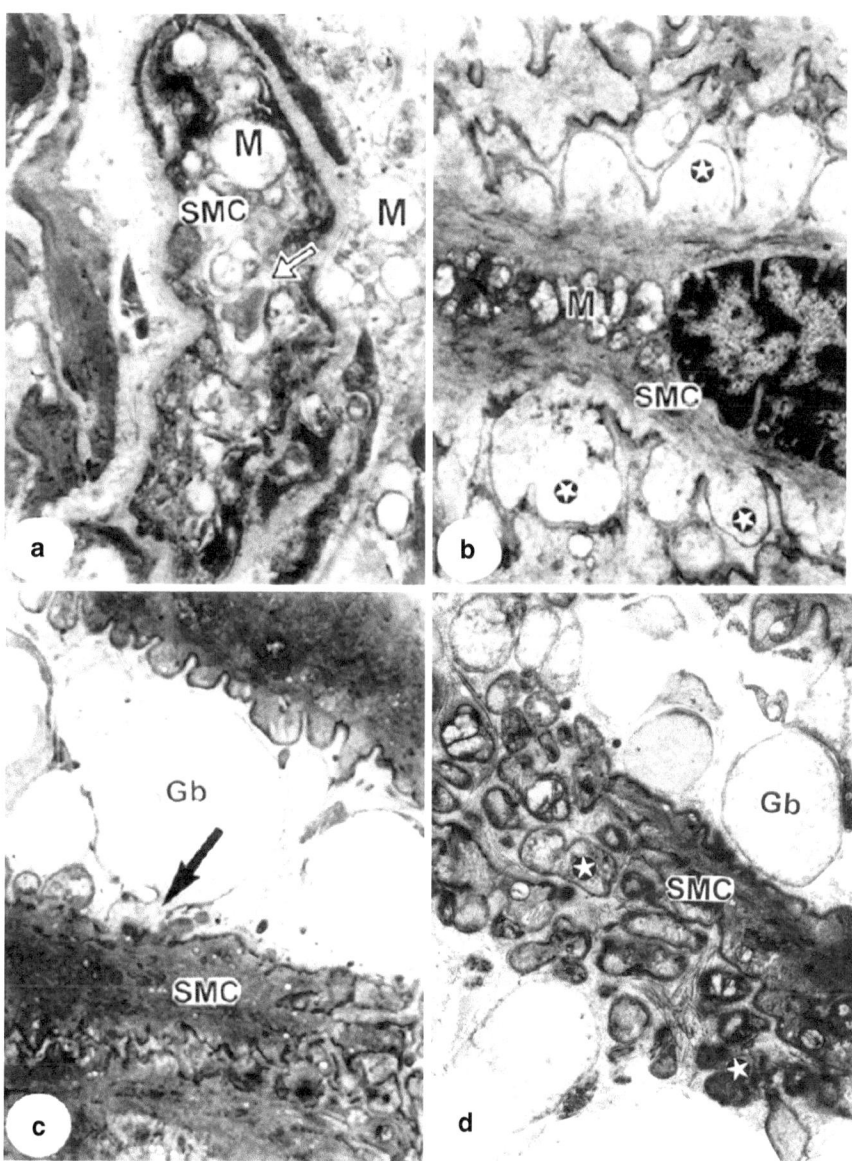

Fig. 2.8 Representative ultrastructural micrographs for SMCs in a LEP of EA/TEF. (**a**) Degenerated SMC showing mitochondrial vacuolation (M) and the presence of myelin figures (arrow) (magnification 15,882×). (**b**) A SMC showing mitochondrial vacuolation (M) and bulging of the cytoplasm into large electrolucent membrane bound-structures (stars) (magnification 13,333×). (**c**) A SMC showing large electrolucent ghost bodies (GB) with a narrow stalk (arrow) (magnification 8269×). (**d**) A fragmented SMC (stars) with formation of ghost bodies (Gb) (magnification 10,400×)

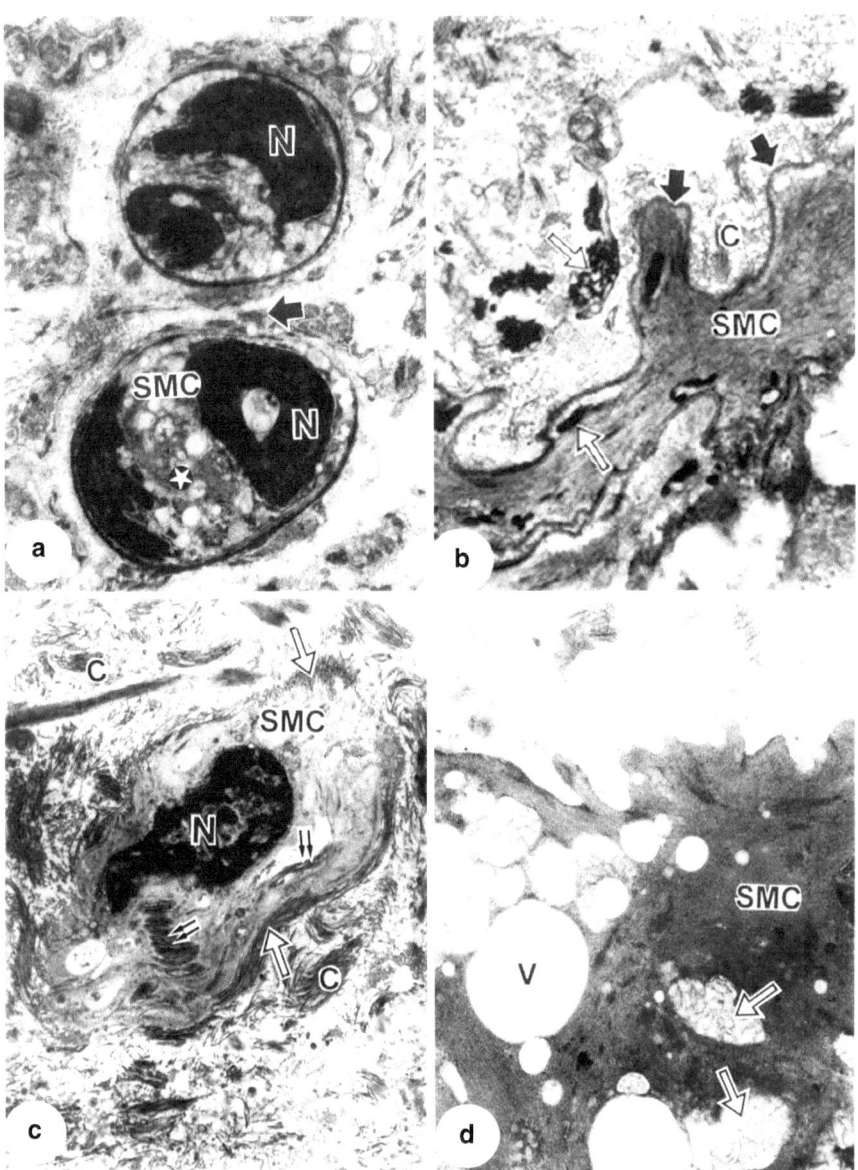

Fig. 2.9 Representative ultrastructural micrographs for SMCs in a LEP of ET/TEF. (**a**) Two SMC apoptotic bodies containing parts of pyknotic nuclei (N) and vacuolated cytoplasm (star) (magnification 17,037×). (**b**) A SMC appeared to extend pseudopodia-like projections (arrows) around collagen fibers (**c**) (magnification 13,600×). (**c**) A SMC containing engulfed collagen fibers (arrows). The inset showing engulfed collagen fibers at a higher magnification (magnification 7333×). (**d**) A SMC showing autophagic vacuoles containing lysed collagen fibers (arrows) and vacuolated mitochondria (M) (magnification 19,200×)

was discovered that delayed maturity in TEF/EA cases and lower density of ICC existed suggesting esophageal dysmotility pathogenesis often seen in such scenarios. Initially, Cajal [15] presented a description of the ICC. The role they play as intestinal pacemakers was reported after ten decades by Maeda et al. [16]. In Midrio et al. study [9], there were variations in the ICC quantity between atretic esophagi and controls. Additionally, an altered ICC morphology alongside the decline in quantity, blocked in EA patients, from forming ICC networks required for relevant motility [17]. The authors found a significant quantity of a cranio-caudal ICC distribution in EA and control cases within the proximal pouch and upper esophagus compared to fistula and distal esophagus. Therefore, the EA distal esophagus remains with very low neuronal cell concentration resulting in impaired peristalsis and defective ICC maturation. TEM analysis proved the results gathered by immunohistochemistry. The ICC controls revealed typical characteristics and feature correlations with nerve endings and muscle cells whereas those for atretic upper esophagus exhibited immaturity with features that resemble fibroblasts. Such atretic esophagus ICC are indeed c-kit negative and might justify the absence of c-kit positive cells as immunohistochemistry highlighted [15]. The EA rat model showed that the left vagus joined the right vagus nerve after the bifurcation of the trachea and the lower esophagus lacked any esophageal plexus [18]. Moreover, a significant reduction in the cell body per ganglion, ganglia, and verve plexus density, existed [18]. In humans, a lower neural tissue fraction existed within the Auerbach plexus layer in the atretic esophagus than in controls; this was clearer within the lower esophagus [19]. Moreover, there were significant hypoganglionosis alongside deficient immature ganglion cell distribution as well as some nerve fibers within the EA proximal end [20, 21]. Li et al. [8], examined the side of fistula within TEF/EA by immunohistochemistry and TEM and discovered abnormal dysplasia of myenteric nerve plexus and imbalanced neurotransmitter release with increased inhibitory neuropeptide expression (nitric oxide and vasoactive intestinal polypeptide).

References

1. Hokama A, Myers NA, Kent M, Campell PE, Chow CW. Esophageal atresia with tracheo-esophageal fistula. A histopathologic study. Pediatr Surg Int. 1986;1:117–21. https://doi.org/10.1007/BF00166872.
2. Merei J, Kotsios C, Hutson JM, Hasthorpe S. Histopathologic study of esophageal atresia and tracheoesophageal fistula in an animal model. J Pediatr Surg. 1997;32:12–4. https://doi.org/10.1016/S0022-3468(97)90081-6.
3. Dutta HK, Mathur M, Bhatnagar V. A histopathological study of esophageal atresia and tracheoesophageal fistula. J Pediatr Surg. 2000;35:438–41. https://doi.org/10.1016/S0022-3468(00)90209-4.
4. Ibrahim AHM, Al Malki TA. Congenital esophageal stenosis associated with esophageal atresia. In: Till H, Thomson M, Foker J, Holcomb III G, Khan K, editors. Esophageal and gastric disorders in infancy and childhood. Berlin: Springer; 2017. p. 113–23. https://doi.org/10.1007/978-3-642-11202-7_131.

5. Al-Shraim MM, Ibrahim AHM, Al Malki TA, Morad N. Histopathologic profile of esophageal atresia and tracheoesophageal fistula. Ann Pediatr Surg. 2014;10:1–6. https://doi.
   org/10.1097/01.XPS.0000438124.55523.06.
6. Davies MRQ. Anatomy of the extrinsic motor nerve supply to mobilized segments of the
   esophagus disrupted by dissection during repair of esophageal atresia with distal fistula. Br J
   Pediatr Surg. 1996;83:1268–70. https://doi.org/10.1046/j.1365-2168.1996.02337.x.
7. Al-Shraim M, Eid R, Musalam A, Radad K, Ibrahim A, Al-Malki T. Ultrastructural changes of
   the smooth muscle in esophageal atresia. Ultrastruct Pathol. 2015;39(6):413–8. https://doi.org
   /10.3109/01913123.2015.106913.
8. LI K, Zheng S, Xiao X, Wang Q, Zhou Y, Chen L, et al. The structural characteristics and
   expression of neuropeptides in the esophagus of patients with congenital esophageal atresia and tracheoesophageal fistula. J Pediatr Surg. 2007;42:1433–8. https://doi.org/10.1016/j.
   jpedsurg.2007.03.050.
9. Midrio P, Faussone-Pellegrini MS, Vannucchi MG, Flake AW. Gastroschisis in the rat model is
   associated with a delayed maturation of intestinal pacemaker cells and smooth muscle cells. J
   Pediatr Surg. 2004;39:1541–7. https://doi.org/10.1016/j.jpedsurg.2004.06.017.
10. Vanderwinden J, Liu H, Menu R, Conreur JL, De Laet MH, Vanderhaeghen JJ. The pathology
    of infantile hypertrophic pyloric stenosis after healing. J Pediatr Surg. 1996;31:1530–4. https://
    doi.org/10.1016/S0022-3468(96)90171-2.
11. Jeng YM, Mao TL, Hsu WM, Huang SF, Hsu HC. Congenital interstitial cell of Cajal hyper-
    plasia with neuronat intestinal dysplasia. Am J Surg Pathol. 2000;24:1568–72.
12. Taniquchi K, Matsuura KTK, Matsuoka T, Nakatani H, Nakaton T, Furuya Y, et al. A mor-
    phological study of the pacemaker cells of the aganglionic intestine in Hirschsprung's dis-
    ease utilizing Is/Is model mice. Med Mol Morphol. 2005;38:123–9. https://doi.org/10.1007/
    s00795-004-0283-y.
13. Midrio P, Alaggio R, Strojna A, Gamba P, Giacomelli L, Pizzi S, et al. Reduction of inter-
    stitial cells of Cajal in esophageal atresia. JPGN. 2010;51(5):610–7. https://doi.org/10.1097/
    MPG.0b013e3181dd9d40.
14. Yamataka A, Ohshiro K, Kobayashi H, Lane GJ, Yamataka T, Fujiwara T, et al. Abnormal
    distribution of intestinal pacemaker (c-kit-positive) cells in an infant with chronic idio-
    pathic intestinal pseudoobstruction. J Pediatr Surg. 1998;33:859–62. https://doi.org/10.1016/
    S0022-3468(98)90660-1.
15. Cajal SR. Sur les ganglions et plexus nerveux de l' intestine. C R Soc Biol (Paris).
    1893;45:217–23.
16. Maeda H, Yamataka A, Nishikawa S, Yoshinaga K, Kobayashi S, Nishi K, et al. Requirement
    of c-kit for development of intestinal pacemaker system. Development. 1992;116:369–75.
17. Sanders KM, Ward SM. Interstitial cells of Cajal- a new perspective on smooth muscle func-
    tion. J Physiol. 2006;576:721–6. https://doi.org/10.1113/jphysiol.2006.115279.
18. Qi BQ, Uemura S, Farmer P, Myers NA, Huston JM. Intrinsic innervation of the esophagus
    in fetal rats with esophageal atresia. Pediatr Surg Int. 1999;15:2–7. https://doi.org/10.1007/
    s003830050499.
19. Nakazato Y, Landing BH, Wells TR. Abnormal Auerbach plexus in the esophagus and
    stomach of patients with esophageal atresia and tracheoesophageal fistula. J Pediatr Surg.
    1986;21:831–7.
20. Boleken M, Demirbilek S, Kirimiloglu H, Hanmaz T, Yucesan S, Celbis O, Uzun I. Reduced
    neuronal innervation in the distal end of the proximal esophageal atretic segment in cases of
    esophageal atresia with distal fistula. World J Surg. 2007;31:1512–7. https://doi.org/10.1007/
    s00268-007-9070-y.
21. Qi BQ, Merei JM, Farmer B, Hasthorpe S, Myers NA, Beasley SW, Hutson JM. The vagus and
    recurrent laryngeal nerves in the rodent experimental model of esophageal atresia. J Pediatr
    Surg. 1997;32:1580–6. https://doi.org/10.1016/S0022.3468(97)90457-7.

Chapter 3
Etiology of Motility Disorders in EA and CES

The esophageal dysfunction etiology in CES cases following EA repair is not only unknown but complex as well. It might be as a result of EA or CES independently or combined. An acquired esophageal dysmotility origin was suggested. Extensive esophageal segment denervation and mobilization could aggravate motility disorders and reflux [1]. Preoperative documentation of normal peristaltic activity was shown within the proximal esophagus in two patients with EA but without fistula. Postoperatively, one patient exhibited a pattern of disturbed motility [2]. Motility dysfunction might be attributed to vagal damage through dissection during EA repair [3]. Serious motor disability has a correlation with extensive mobilization of the pouch [4].

A congenital source for esophageal motility disorders following EA repair was suggested. Romeo et al. [5] has preoperatively recorded disturbed motility among EA patients. Moreover, motility disorders have been found in isolated TEF without EA patients [6]. Motility disorders were not evident after esophageal transection and anastomosis [7]. Limited histological research has been undertaken within the literature to record the congenital source of esophageal dysmotility following successful EA repair. Animal models [8–10] and autopsy patients [11, 12] were used in many of the studies that were undertaken. Abnormal Auerbach plexus was discovered within the stomach and esophagus in five EA and TEF autopsy patients. Within the distal esophagus, the plexus was abnormally looser and to some extent within the stomach fundus and proximal esophagus. The size of the ganglia was unusually larger. The strata of the smooth muscle were found to be normal [12]. In other studies [8, 11, 13, 14], Tracheo-bronchial remnants (TBR) with or without cartilage were described. TBR with cartilage, seromucus glands and ciliated pseudo-stratified columnar epithelia alongside irregular smooth muscle fiber were observed within distal esophagus sections as illustrated in Figs. 2.1 and 2.2. Seromucus glands were observed among lower esophageal pouch muscle bundles that cause significant distortion. Additionally, there was documentation for abnormal mucus glands that cause muscle distortion. The shift from fistula towards normal esophageal histology

© Springer Nature Switzerland AG 2019
A. Ibrahim, T. Al-Malki, *Congenital Esophageal Stenosis*,
https://doi.org/10.1007/978-3-030-10782-6_3

occurs at variable distances from the fistula source and might extend downwards towards the cardiac end of the esophagus [8, 11, 13]. Moreover, surgical samples from the upper and lower pouches revealed histological image aligned to FMD as illustrated in Fig. 2.3 [13, 14].

Singarm et al. [15] investigated the histological and immunohistochemical characteristics of FMD CES in two adults. Compared to three controls, CES esophagi exhibited neutrophil infiltration within the myenteric planes without collagen increments. NADPH-diaphorase histochemistry exhibited a considerable decline of circular muscle fibers and myenteric nitrinergic neurons. In particular, the overall nitric oxide (NO) inhibitory innervations' absence might constitute an essential mechanism within the esophagus aperistalsis and stenosis pathogenesis in the disorder.

In humans [16–18] and in models of Adriamycin fetal rat [9, 10], neuropeptides can be considered abnormal, particularly in the atretic esophagus. The cell body per ganglia immune-stained by substance P (SP), vasoactive intestinal peptide (VIP), or neuron specific enolase (NSE), coupled with the ganglia and nerve plexus density decreased significantly within TEF/EA fetuses. Therefore, considerable intramural nervous component abnormalities of the TEF/EA rat esophagus exist, involving inhibitory (VIP-labelled) and excitatory (SP-labelled) intramural nerves that might be attributing to TEF/EA esophageal dysmotility [9]; the circumferential distribution of myenteric plexus neurons within the rat model's atretic esophagus decreased by 50%. The nearly-complete nerve tissue ring along the myenteric plexus plane was substituted with nerve tissue clusters within the atretic esophagus. Arguably, the esophageal dysmotility observed in EA [19] could be attributed to the abnormal nerve tissue distribution within the atretic esophagus. Qi et al., applying a similar model demonstrated that vagus nerve produced fewer branches within the esophagus and adopted abnormal pathway at the lower esophagus level [20]. Boleken et al. [16] investigated the proximal esophageal atretic segment distal ends of neonates subjected to TEF/EA repair for intrinsic neuronal innervations. Their findings revealed a deficiency in terms of distributed nerve fibers and ganglion cells. The esophagus' abnormal and insufficient neuronal innervations might have a correlation with EA esophageal dysmotility. Deficient glial cell line-derived neurotrophic factor (GDNF) expression might play a crucial role within the abnormal or defective atretic esophageal segment's neuronal innervations [16]. Likewise, Li et al. [17] examined the structural features as well as the neuropeptide cohort expression within the samples collected from the TEF/EA patients' lower esophagus fistulous end. Their findings showed neurotransmitter imbalances within the nerve vesicles, excessive expression of some neuropeptides such as VIP, abnormal nerve plexus intrinsic dysplasia, and an abnormal intrinsic innervated esophagus characterized by VIP and nitric oxide synthase (NOS), which might be the cause of post-operative esophageal dysfunction [17].

Pederiva et al. investigated the intrinsic esophageal innervation in children having isolated EA with samples from the distal and proximal esophageal segments. There were larger ganglia and denser fibrilar networks compared to those for controls [18].

Zuccarello et al. [21] investigated the structures of intramural ganglions within EA; they employed 12 esophageal samples for histochemical and histological studies. The atretic components revealed qualitative and quantitative variations with sparsely distributed nervous tissues within the distal samples compared to that for proximal samples and controls. From a histological perspective, the atretic segments featured disorganized muscle bundles containing fibrosis within upper esophageal pouch (UEP), edema, and hyper-plastic lining epithelia. Notably, disarranged muscularis propria and muscularis mucosa, abnormal sub-mucosal elastic fibers, muscular and mucosal hypoplasia characterized the lower esophageal pouch (LEP). From an immunohisto-chemical viewpoint, Actin-A studies revealed fragmented and disorganized muscle bundles that reached the baseline of the epithelia and muscularis mucosa segmental agenesis. There was reduction of Anti-A immunostaining within the UEP smooth muscle bundles and within the LEP, it was weaker. Regarding S-100, the UEP indicated lesser ganglion cells within the myenteric plexus whereas the immunoreactivity increased for S-100 compared to that for control. The LEP exhibited negligible tiny immature cells containing less significant immunostaining compared to that for UEP. With regard to neuro-filament (NF), a diffused weak expression of immuno-staining at the myenteric region of the two atretic esophageal segments, existed. In some instances, the immune-reactivity of NF was missing within the LEP. Regarding Peripherin (P), the immune-reactivity was less significant within the UEP myenteric ganglion cells compared to those for LEP. Notably, Neuron Specific Enolase (NSE) indicated a fragile cytoplasmic positivity within the distal and proximal segments. Chromogranin A (CgnA) indicated the presence of a significant positive immunoreactivity within the UEP compared to that for lower. Zuccarello et al. [21] concluded that segments of atretic esophagi particularly the lower ones containing P-immunostaining indicated the existence of neuroblasts (immature neuronal cells), whereas with Cgn A immunoreactivity, granin deficiency with subsequent changed neurotransmitter activity release was found. The above findings reveal a time-overrun in the organization of myenteric plexus and neuronal differentiation, which might account for the motility disorder within TEF/EA. Furthermore, the results complement the view that histomorphological changes of the nervous and muscular elements in the esophageal walls could contribute towards esophageal dysmotility among patients following TEF/EA surgeries [21].

Kawahara et al. [22] examined the motor function in four isolated CES cases. One case was membranous, one with TBR whereas two cases constituted FMD. Esophagogram revealed swift clearance within the membranous case whereas a contrast proximal stasis existed to the distal esophageal narrowing within the two FMD cases and TBR case. Three patients exhibited exposure to pathologic acid through pH tracking despite the absence of esophagitis evidence through endoscopy. Manometry indicated peristaltic waves in the membranous case and synchronous esophageal contractions in FMD and TBR cases. The pressure of lower esophageal sphincter (LES) was about 20 mmHg. LES relaxation induced by swallowing was complete within the membranous whereas in the remaining three cases, it was incomplete. The authors posited that TBR and FMD CES are dominated by gastro esophageal reflux (GER) and impaired esophageal motility. Synchronous contractions observed within TBR and FMD patients might be linked to nitric oxide's abnormal innervations. The manometric data within CES among children cited by Pittsburgh cohort revealed segmental aperistaltic region at the stenosis level with local reduced pliability. The inferior and superior sphincters had a normal response to swallowing [22]. A manometric investigation within 12 CES cases revealed another high pressure zone (HPZ) besides the LES discovered in nine patients. The additional pressure region vanished following treatment [23].

Cheng [24] reported an achalasia-like esophageal dysmotility within a 14-year-old boy following successful TEF/EA repair in the neonatal periods. This was proved through clinical, manometric, and radiological studies. The manometric characteristics constituted a cardiac sphincter with a length of 2 cm and a high pressure exceeding 40 mmHg with aperistalsis within the esophageal body coupled with the cardiac sphincter inability to relax following a swallow. The condition reacted properly to Hiller's myotomy [24].

Kawahara et al. [25] reported on the importance of videomanometry for examining pediatric esophageal motor diseases in four TEF/EA postoperative cases alongside one isolated distal CES case due to TBR-mimicking achalasia. Such cases often exhibited impaired esophageal transit in defective esophageal peristaltic contractions. Video fluoroscopic images within EA cases indicated significant contrast stasis within the body of esophagus. The distal esophagus indicated low-amplitude peristaltic contractions in two cases, no contractions within one case, and synchronous contractions with low amplitude in a single case. Overall, the authors posited that impaired esophageal transit was triggered by defective luminal closures particularly within the middle esophagus in deglutition; however, not through LES malfunction.

Video fluoroscopy for the CES case revealed contrast stasis within the distal dilated esophagus with narrowing at the lower esophageal end mimicking achalasia. Manometry revealed swallow—induced LES relaxation with low amplitude synchronous contractions all over the esophageal body. Topographic plotting indicated swallow-induced LES relaxation as well as the lack of second and third segments for the sequential pressure event chain implying that the pattern of LES motor is incompatible with esophageal achalasia. The defective luminal closure resulting in an impaired esophageal transit was extended all over the esophageal body.

Lemoine et al. [26] utilized high-resolution esophageal Manometry (HREM) to classify motility trends in 40 pediatric patients with repaired EA and contrasted the trends against symptomatology. Seven patients only (17.5%) were found to be asymptomatic; however, in all patients, HREM outcomes were abnormal. Notably, HREM experienced three different patterns of esophageal motility. Aperistalsis was observed in 15 patients (38%) with GER disease related symptom. Pressurization was observed in 15% (6 patients). Distal contractions were observed in 47% (19 patients) only in type C EA.

Most distal contraction group cases featured segregated middle third esophageal contractions (containing high distal and proximal trough). The proximal trough length (transitional zone) is found to cause dysphagia in adults if it exceeds 5 cm. Pediatrics is yet to quantify it. In patients with EA with 'distal contraction 'the median transitional zone was 7.6 cm and the shortest was 4.5 cm. Indeed, it could be supposed that a long transitional zone in a child must have symptoms. The cohort of pressurization trend has a lake of an organized peristalsis and denotes neuropathic discoordination of longitudinal and circular muscle contraction. The aperistalsis cohort was encountered predominantly within cases of leakage and long gap. Esophagitis was discovered in children with pressurization and aperistalsis cohorts.

Rayyan et al. [27] claimed that esophageal dysmotility constituted the main cause of dysphagia in EA. The problem is aggravated when a structural pathology like esophageal stricture or CES is superimposed on the underlying disordered motility. Both manometry and esophagogram are utilized for evaluating the esophagogastric junction (EGJ) and esophageal motor function and anatomy. Manometry has served as the diagnostic choice tool. In the past 10 years, high resolution manometry (HRM) has acquired recognition as the diagnostic tool for a variety of motility trends. Indeed, such approaches (manometry and esophagogram) could fail to link an esophageal motor disorder with symptoms'. The latest technique known as pressure flow analysis (PFA) concurrently integrates manometry measurements and acquired impedance and utilizes a combined analysis of such recordings to obtain metrics of quantitative pressure flow [28]. Such metrics enable identification of the correlation between symptomatology, motor patterns, and bolus flow by integrating data on the resistance of bolus flow and bolus transit. Dysphagia symptoms coupled with increased bolus passage perception might show enhanced resistance towards flow at GEJ or retarded esophageal propulsion.

Additionally, Rayyan et al. [27] posited that esophageal dysmotility etiology is still debatable. They categorized motility disorders into primary, secondary, or tertiary. Primary motility disorders are triggered by abnormal esophageal muscle growth or intrinsic or extrinsic esophageal innervations. The interstitial Cajal cells that are intestinal pacemakers facilitating intestinal peristalsis propagation and rhythmicity are indeed deficient in EA patients [28]. GER and surgery is the cause of secondary motility disorders. Structural pathology emanating from GER peptic strictures, CES, anastomotic strictures is the cause of tertiary motility disorders [29, 30].

Diagnostic Tools to Investigate Dysphagia in EA [27]

Esophagogram constitutes the first diagnostic tool for investigating dysphagia for patients subjected to surgery for EA and is capable of diagnosing strictures alongside other functional disorders through dynamic studies. Nevertheless, manometry constitutes the preferred diagnostic tool for diagnosing esophageal motor disorders. HRM provides new viewpoints in identifying motility trends. There is improved reliability of modified equipment, increased sensor resolution as well as transition from perfused towards solid-state sensors and smaller catheter diameters. Such technical advances enabled pressure recording visualization not solely as tracing of lines but as esophageal pressure topography (EPT) clouse plots. Based upon the EPT metrics, obtained from the plots, various motor function patterns are identified. Such trends are categorized into a diagnostic algorithm namely the Chicago classification diagnostic algorithm that offers normative guidelines and values for assessing esophageal motor functions [31]. Such HRM motor trends lacked clear motor pattern trend interplay with the symptoms. The HRM impedance was unveiled but significantly failed to offer the anticipated diagnostic gains and to enable definition of a relationship with the clinical symptoms [26].

There may be insensitivity of the technologies applied, an absence of a combined manometry analytical method as well as impedance recording. Normal esophageal clearance can also be attained with abnormal motility pattern [32]. PFA was unveiled to enable combined analysis of simultaneously recorded bolus flow and esophageal motility. Notably, the PFA metrics is beneficial to assess non-obstructive dysphagia, [33] post fundoplication dysphagia [34] and allow for the separation of dysphagia-free patients from dysphagia patients [35]. The PFA could compute the impedance ratio (IR), the pressure-flow index (PFI), and pressure-flow metrics. The PFI constitutes a composite bolus pressurization measure compared to flow whereas the impedance ratio (IR) refers to the measurement of the degree of bolus clearance failure. Moreover, the pressure flow matrix that combines IR and PFI could be determined as well [34]. The latter is capable of separating dysphagia patients due to abnormal clearance of bolus from GEJ-based abnormal bolus resistance.

Rayyan et al. [27] review of the topic reiterated that dysphagia clinical diagnosis in EA patients is dependent upon clinical symptoms, radiologic evaluation and low-resolution manometric. However, modern diagnosis features HRM supported with measurements of impedance to evaluate the correlation between bolus clearance and esophageal motor function. Through the novel PFA technique as the combined manometric analysis method coupled with impedance measurements might be clinically essential for differentiating bolus outflow disorder patients from impaired GEJ relaxation patients. Pressure flow matrix constitutes a potentially objective platforms of making rational therapeutic choices regarding whether bolus clearance should be improved pharmacologically or GEJ flow resistance within symptomatic EA patients should be reduced. Additionally, PFA could assist to forecast postoperative dysphagia among patients subjected to fundoplication [27]. Dysphagia of CES and/or EA cases are approached in our institute by a consultation to the ENT and pediatric teams. We depend on the clinical picture, contrast upper GI studies, results of histology taken from the tips of esophageal pouches during primary repair and upper gastrointestinal endoscopy. If histology shows CES then we expect motility disorder and/or anastomotic stricture. FMD has a better response towards dilatation whereas TBR might need resection. Interestingly, one of our TBR cases reacted well towards dilatation; however, there was significant esophageal body dysmotility that improved following lower esophageal myectomy, gastrostomy and Thal fundoplication.

Myectomy indicated normal histology (Fig. 3.1a–c). The surgery is aimed at having a feeding gastrostomy, to avert GER and to acquire a sample of histology from the lower esophagus. There was weakened propulsive wave that influenced

Fig. 3.1 (**a**) TBR with cartilage obtained from the tip of the lower esophageal pouch during primary repair. (**b**) Initial normal barium swallow and meal. (**c**) Photo from video fluoroscopy with major dysmotility after 1 month with failure of passage of the contrast distally for more than 5 min. Barium swallow and meal after fundoplication and lower esophageal myectomy showed motility improvement

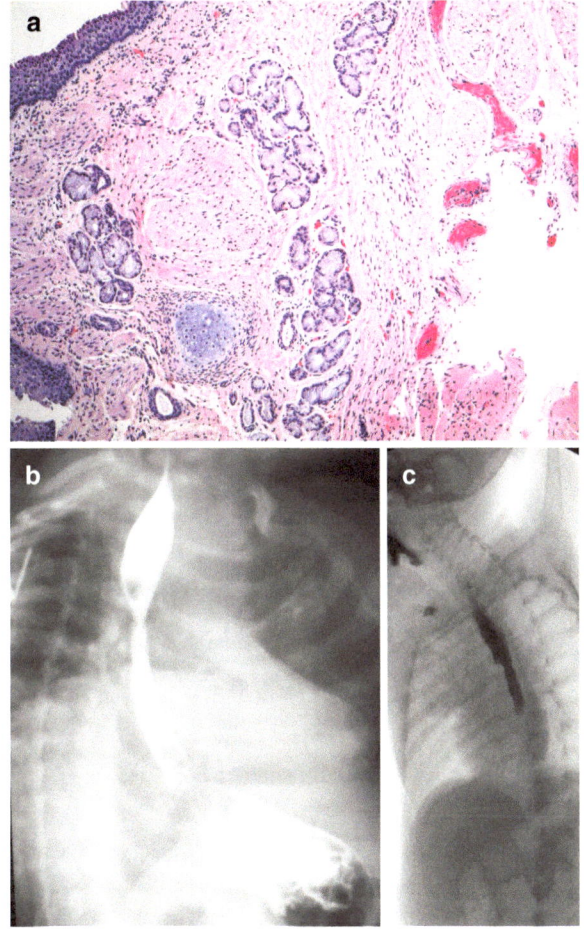

bolus flow. There was no low-resolution manometry at the time. The 24-h reflux index has the North America and Europe approval as the most sensitive and specific GERD predictor. One major problem is its incapacity to identify non-acid reflux. Multichannel intra-luminal impedance is capable of evaluating liquid direction and velocity as well as the flow of gas via the esophagus. CES cases with EA might influence the anastomotic region or distal to it. The stenotic region could be influenced by FMD or TBR forms of CES. The stenosis may be refractory to dilatation, particularly when GERD and dysmotility exist. The dysmotility, GER, and stenosis triad might constitute a complex scenario to treat. Antireflux measures and dilatation might fail to overcome this complex scenario. The patient is often in a bad general condition. Malnourishment and FTT exist because of dysphagia and intolerance to feeds. There is a serious respiratory compromise with repetitive aspiration pneumonia and chest infections, and the patients often needs endotracheal ventilation. Following partial fundoplication (posterior or anterior), alongside gastrostomy accompanied by dilatation constitute our management plan, which is adopted in such complex situation. In the event that dilatation is not successful, then resection and anastomosis is needed. Postoperatively, some dilatation sessions might be needed a well [36].

References

1. Orringer MB, Kirsch MM, Sloan H. Long term esophageal function following repair of esophageal atresia. Ann Surg. 1977;186:436–43.
2. Shono T, Suita S, Arima T, Handa N, Ishhlii K, Hirose R, et al. Motility function of the esophagus before primary anastomosis in esophageal atresia. J Pediatr Surg. 1993;28:673–6.
3. Davies MRQ. Anatomy of the extrinsic motor nerve supply to mobilized segments of the esophagus disrupted by dissection during repair of esophageal atresia with distal fistula. Br J Pediatr Surg. 1996;83:1268–70. https://doi.org/10.1046/j.1365-2168.1996.02337.x.
4. Cavallaro S, Pineschi A, Freni G, Cortese MG, Bardini T. Feeding troubles following delayed primary repair of esophageal atresia with distal fistula Eur. J Pediatr Surg. 1992;2:73–7. https://doi.org/10.1055/s-2008-1063406.
5. Romeo JG, Zuccarello B, Proietto F, Romeo C. Disorders of the esophageal motor activity in atresia of the esophagus. J Pediatr Surg. 1987;22:120–4. https://doi.org/10.1016/s0022-3468(87)80425-6.
6. Johnston P, Newlin Hustings N. Congenital tracheoesophageal fistula without esophageal atresia. Am J Surg. 1966;112:233–40. https://doi.org/10.1016/0002-9610(66)90014-6.
7. Haller JA, Brooker AF, Talbert J, Baghdassarian O, Vanhoutte J, et al. Esophageal function following resection: studies in newborn puppies. Ann Thorac Surg. 1966;2:180–7.
8. Merei J, Kotsios C, Hutson JM, Hasthorpe S. Histopathologic study of esophageal atresia and tracheoesophageal fistula in an animal model. J Pediatr Surg. 1997;32:12–4. https://doi.org/10.1016/S0022-3468(97)90081-6.
9. Cheng W, Bishop AE, Spitz L, Bolak JM. Abnormalities of neuropeptides and neural markers in the esophagus of fetal rats with adriamycin-induced esophageal atresia. J Pediatr Surg. 1997;32:1420–3. https://doi.org/10.1016/S0022-3468(97)90552-2.
10. Qi BQ, Uemura S, Farmer P, Myers NA, Huston JM. Intrinsic innervation of the esophagus in fetal rats with esophageal atresia. Pediatr Surg Int. 1999;15:2–7. https://doi.org/10.1007/s00383005049.
11. Hokama A, Myers NA, Kent M, Campell PE, Chow CW. Esophageal atresia with tracheoesophageal fistula. A histopathologic study. Pediatr Surg Int. 1986;1:117–21. https://doi.org/10.1007/BF00166872.
12. Nakazato Y, Landing BH, Wells TR. Abnormal Auerbach plexus in the esophagus and stomach of patients with esophageal atresia and tracheoesophageal fistula. J Pediatr Surg. 1986;21:831–7.
13. Ibrahim AH, Al Malki TA, Hamza AF, Bahnasy AF. Congenital esophageal stenosis associated with esophageal atresia: new concepts. Pediatr Surg Int. 2007;23:533–7. https://doi.org/10.1007/s00383-007-1927-5.
14. Al-Shraim MM, Ibrahim AHM, Al Malki TA, Morad N. Histopathologic profile of esophageal atresia and tracheoesophageal fistula. Ann Pediatr Surg. 2014;10:1–6. https://doi.org/10.1097/01.XPS.0000438124.55523.06.
15. Singarm C, Sweet MA, Gaumnitz EA, Cameron A. Peptidergic and nitrinergic denervation in congenital esophageal stenosis. Gastroenterology. 1995;109:275–81. https://doi.org/10.1016/0016-5085(95)90294-5.

16. Boleken M, Demirbilek S, Kirimiloglu H, Hanmaz T, Yucesan S, Celbis O, Uzun I. Reduced neuronal innervation in the distal end of the proximal esophageal atretic segment in cases of esophageal atresia with distal fistula. World J Surg. 2007;31:1512–7. https://doi.org/10.1007/s00268-007-9070-y.

17. Li K, Zheng S, Xiao X, Wang Q, Zhon Y, Chen L. The structural characteristics and expression of neuropeptides in the esophagus of patients with congenital esophageal atresia and tracheoesophageal fistula. J Pediatr Surg. 2007;42:1433–8. https://doi.org/10.1016/j.jpedsurg.2007.03.050.

18. Pederiva F, Burgos E, Francicol I, Zuccrello B, Martinez L, Tovar JA. Intrinsic esophageal innervation in esophageal atresia without fistula. Pediatr Surg Int. 2008;24:95–100. https://doi.org/10.1007/s00383-007-2032-5.

19. Cheng W, Bishop AE, Spitz L, Polak JM. Abnormal enteric nerve morphology in atretic esophagus of fetal rats with Adriamycin induced esophageal atresia. Pediatr Surg Int. 1999;15:8–10. https://doi.org/10.1007/s003830050500.

20. Qi BQ, Merei JM, Farmer D, Hasthorpe S, Myers NA, Beasley SW, Hutson JM. The vagus and recurrent laryngeal nerves in the rodent experimental model of esophageal atresia. J Pediatr Surg. 1997;32:1580–6. https://doi.org/10.1016/S0022-3468(97)90457-7.

21. Zuccarello B, Spada A, Turiaco N, Parisi S, Francica I, Francica S, et al. Intramural ganglion structures in esophageal atresia: a morphologic and immunohistochemical study. Int J Pediatr. 2009;2009:695837. https://doi.org/10.1155/2009/695837.

22. Kawahara H, Oue T, Okuyama H, Kubota A, Okada A. Esophageal motor function in congenital esophageal stenosis. J Pediatr Surg. 2003;38:1716–9. https://doi.org/10.1016/j.jpedsurg.2003.08.020.

23. Amae S, Nio M, Kamiyama T, Ishii T, Yoshida S, Hayashi Y, et al. Clinical characteristics and management of congenital esophageal stenosis: a report on 14 cases. J Pediatr Surg. 2003;38:565–70. https://doi.org/10.1053/jpsu.2003.50123.

24. Cheng W, Poon KH, Lui VCH, Yong JL, Law S, So KT, Tse K, Tam PKH. Esophageal atresia and achalasia like esophageal dysmotility. J Pediatr Surg. 2004;39:1581–3. https://doi.org/10.1016/j.jpedsurg.2004.06.027.

25. Kawahara H, Kubota A, Okuyama H, Oue T, Tazuke Y, Okada A. The usefulness of video-manometry for studying pediatric esophageal motor disease. J Pediatr Surg. 2004;39:1754–7. https://doi.org/10.1016/j.jpedsurg.2004.08.032.

26. Lemoine C, Aspirot A, Henaff G, Piloquet H, Lévesque D, Faure C. Characterization of esophageal motility following esophageal atresia repair using high-resolution esophageal manometry. JPGN. 2013;56:609–14. https://doi.org/10.1097/MPG.0b013e3182868773.

27. Rayyan M, Alegaert K, Omari T, Rommel N. Dysphagia in children with esophageal atresia: current diagnostic options. Eur J Pediatr Surg. 2015;25(4):326–32. https://doi.org/10.1055/s-0035-1559818.

28. Midrio P, Alaggio R, Strojna A, Gamba P, Giacomelli L, Pizzi S, et al. Reduction of interstitial cells of Cajal in esophageal atresia. JPGN. 2010;51:610–7. https://doi.org/10.1097/MPG.0b013e3181dd9d40.

29. McCann F, Michaud L, Aspirot A, Levesque D, Gottrand F, Faure C. Congenital esophageal stenosis associated with esophageal atresia. Dis Esophagus. 2015;28:211–5. https://doi.org/10.1111/dote.12176.

30. Baird R, Laberge JM, Lévesque D. Anastomotic stricture after esophageal atresia repair: a critical review of recent literature. Eur J Pediatr Surg. 2013;23:204–13. https://doi.org/10.1055/s-0033-1347917.

31. Bredenoord AJ, Fox M, Kahrilas PJ, Pandolfino JE, Schwizer W, Smout AJ, International High Resolution Manometry Working Group. Chicago classification criteria of esophageal motility disorders defined in high resolution esophageal pressure topography. Neurogastroenterol Motil. 2012;24(suppl 1):57–65. https://doi.org/10.1111/j.1365-2982.2011.01834.x.

32. Van Wijk M, Knuppe F, Omari T, DE long J, Benninga M. Evaluation of gastroesophageal functional mechanisms underlying gastro-esophageal reflux in infants and adults born with esophageal atresia. J Pediatr Surg. 2013;48:2496–505. https://doi.org/10.1016/j.jpedsurg2013.07.024.
33. Nguyen NQ, Holloway RH, Smout AJ, Omari TI. Automated impedance manometry analysis detects esophageal motor dysfunction in patients who have non-obstructive dysphagia with normal manometry. Neurogastroenterol Motil. 2013;25(3):238–45, e.164. https://doi.org/10.1111/nmo.12040.
34. Myers JC, Nguyen NQ, Jamieson GG, Van't Hek JE, Ching K, Holloway RH, et al. Susceptibility to dysphagia after fundoplication revealed by novel automated impedance manometry analysis. Neurogastroenterol Motil. 2012;24(9):812–e393. https://doi.org/10.1111/j.1365-2982.2012.01938.x.
35. Rommel N, Van Oudenhove L, Tack J, Omari TI. Automated impedance manometry analysis as a method to assess esophageal function. Neurogastroenterol Motil. 2014;26(5):636–45. https://doi.org/10.1111/nmo.12308.
36. Ibrahim AHM, Bazeed MF, Jamil S, Hamad HA, Abdel Raheem IM, Ashraf I. Management of congenital esophageal stenosis associated with esophageal atresia and its impact on postoperative esophageal stricture. Ann Pediatr Surg. 2016;12:36–4. https://doi.org/10.1097/01.XPS.0000482656.06000.84.

Chapter 4
The Spectrum of CES

The Spectrum of CES

CES represents a wide spectrum of diseases. It can be associated with EA and/or TEF [1] or it can be isolated lesion (not associated with EA). CES associated with EA may affect the anastomotic site or distal to it [1–3]. The lesion can be tracheobronchial remnants (TBR), Fibromuscular disease (FMD) or rarely a membranous disease (MD). The latter may be isolated lesion or associated with EA. It may be a complete diaphragm or a perforated one. CES distal to the anastomotic site may be proximal to the gastroesophageal junction (GEJ) allowing free GER. However, it may involve the GEJ mimicking cardiac achalasia [4]. An isolated CES can affect any part of the esophagus; upper, middle lower esophagus or even the cardiac end.

Fékété et al. [5] defined CES as intrinsic stenosis caused by congenital malformation of the esophageal wall present at birth, although not necessarily symptomatic during the neonatal period. The definition is excellent to describe the intrinsic part of the disease. However, it ignores the intramural membranous part of the disease and the external compression caused for example by vascular rings. We propose a new definition to include all causes of the disease. CES is present at birth, but not essentially symptomatic, due to intra-mural, intrinsic with textural abnormalities or extramural compression resulting in congenital narrowing of the esophagus.

The intrinsic causes involve a type with tracheobronchial remnant (TBR) (Figs. 2.1 and 2.2), another with segmental hypertrophy of the muscularis and diffuse fibrosis of the submucosa (FMD) (Fig. 2.3). The most common type of CES was that of the TBR variety (75%) followed by the FMD (25%) [6]. Terui et al. [7] reported in a systematic review of 144 literatures in 2015 that the frequency was 54% for FMD, 30% for TBR and 16% for the membranous web. These percentages might not be correct. The FMD responds better to balloon dilatation. If dilatation is successful, no histological specimen is available. So, a definitive incidence of subtypes cannot be determined. Also the percentage of each type that will respond to dilatation is not known. It is possible that CES can be multiple. The stenotic area

© Springer Nature Switzerland AG 2019
A. Ibrahim, T. Al-Malki, *Congenital Esophageal Stenosis*,
https://doi.org/10.1007/978-3-030-10782-6_4

may involve the perianastomotic area of EA or even may extend distally to a variable distance [1, 6]. For this reason, we disagree with the statement that CES does not involve the anastomotic site and is always separate from it [8]. However, a distal isolated area of CES separate from the anastomotic site may be present [6, 9]. All the 11 cases reported by Kawahara in 2001 were found to have narrowing between the anastomosis and the gastro esophageal junction; in the mid esophagus in two and in the lower esophagus in nine patients [6]. Most recently [10], the TBR cases were 10 out of 40 (25.0%) while the FMD was 27 out of 40 cases (67.5%). One case had MD together with FMD (2.5%).

In our experience, we had 16 cases of CES associated with EA. Two cases had gastric pull-up due to extension of the TBR from the anastomotic site down to the cardia and are excluded from further studies. Five of 14 cases had FMD and 9 had TBR of which 4 had TBR without cartilage. The FMD affected the anastomotic site in two cases and the distal esophagus in 3 cases all sparing the GEJ. The TBR affected the anastomotic site in 8 cases and one affected the distal esophagus sparing the GEJ. Distal CES that spares the GEJ may have the ominous triad of GER, stricture and dysmotility with all of its sequelae. This situation usually happens in cases of CES associated with EA, the management of which might prove very difficult. This will be discussed in details in the section of treatment of CES.

Isolated CES can affect the esophagus at any site but more frequently in the distal esophagus. If it involves the GEJ, then it will behave like achalasia of the cardia with no possible GER. The differentiation between CES involving the GEJ and achalasia is important because CES, especially TBR type, may not respond to myotomy [4, 11]. The upper dilated esophagus of CES cases shows tertiary contractions unlike the atonic esophagus of achalasia. We had experience with 11 cases treated for isolated CES. Five cases were TBR as proved by resection and histology. Four involved the GEJ and one Down syndrome patient involving the mid esophagus who presented with FB impaction. Six patients were suspected to have FMD who responded to balloon dilatation. One patient had a double lesion in the upper third of the esophagus, a perforated diaphragm and another lower one probably FMD (Fig. 4.1). Two distal esophageal (probably FMD) sparing the GEJ. Three patients had distal esophageal involvement mostly FMD lesions involving the GEJ. Double CES lesions have been also reported by others [10, 12, 13]. CES has been documented in families [14, 15] and in adults [16]. Such cases are actually mild forms of the disease that may be asymptomatic or discovered accidentally or have mild symptoms and signs that is tolerated by the patient for a long period.

CES Associated Congenital Anomalies

The incidence of other anomalies associated with CES is reported to be 17–33% [17]. These anomalies include EA with or without TEF, N-type fistula, cardiac anomalies, intestinal atresia, midgut malrotation, anorectal malformations, hypospadias, malformation of the head and face, limb anomalies and chromosomal anomalies [5].

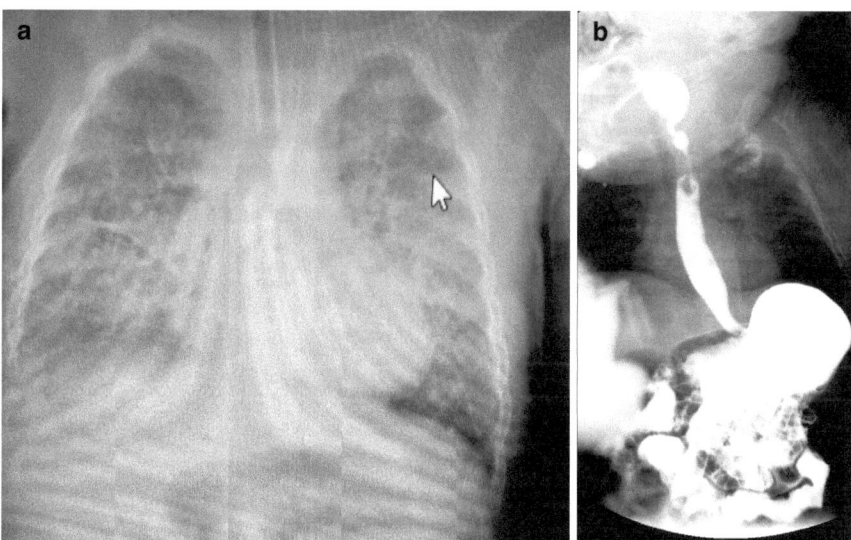

Fig. 4.1 A 20 days old female with intolerance to oral feeds with recurrent aspiration pneumonia. (**a**) Chest X-ray showing severe pneumonia. (**b**) Barium swallow showed a double lesion of upper esophageal CES which responded well to 3 sessions of dilatations

Kawahara et al. reported that 14% of their patients with EA had associated CES [6]. This high incidence was further supported by our team in 2007 and 2015 [1, 2]. Due to this high incidence of this association, it is possible that associated anomalies of EA may be also present in cases of CES. It is reported that 50% of infants born with an esophageal atresia have at least one associated anomaly. The most common are cardiac, genitourinary, gastrointestinal, vertebral/skeletal and genetic defects (trisomy 21, 18 and 13) [19]. Partial or complete VACTERL syndrome (vertebral, anorectal, cardiac, tracheoesophageal, renal and limb anomalies) may also be present. McCann reported 17 cases of CES associated with EA. Four had VACTERL syndrome, two had trisomy 21, two imperforated anuses, two VSD and one duodenal atresia [18]. Vasudevan et al. [20] reported 6 patients with CES. Four patients had associated anomalies. One patient had EA/TEF, Aortopulmonary window, atrial situs solitus, left superior vena cava to coronary sinus, left pelvocaliectasis, L6 hemivertebra and right inguinal hernia. The second had EA/TEF and tracheomalacia. The third had N-type TEF and the fourth had EA, duodenal atresia, duodenal web, VSD and ASD [20]. Associated imperforate anus, cardiac anomalies, duodenal atresia and Currarino triad have been reported in cases of CES associated with EA/TEF [12].

Most recently, Suzuhigashi et al. in a 10-year multicenter study of 40 consecutive cases of CES in Kyushu area in Japan found a high associated anomalies reaching up to 52.5% [10]. There were 8 patients in that study with associated EA (20.0%). A total of 34 associated anomalies were recognized in 21 patients. Nine patients had two associated anomalies, and two patients had three associated anomalies. Down's syndrome was recognized in two patients. The congenital associated anomalies included: gastrointestinal in 13 (EA Gross A in 2, Gross C in 6, gastric volvulus in 1, duodenal atresia in 1, malrotation in 1 and imperforate anus in 2), cardiovascular in 5, urogenital in 3, Down's syndrome in 2, and others in 11.

In our experience with 27 cases of CES, 16 patients (59.3%) had associated EA and 11 patients (40.7%) were isolated CES. In total, 12 patients had other associated anomalies. These 12 patients had CP/brain atrophy in 4, ASD in 2, VSD in 3, PDA in 2, Down syndrome in 2, ARM in 1, Fanconi anemia in 1, skeletal anomalies in 1 and thoracic stomach in 1 (Table 4.1).

Sharma et al. [21] reported a case of congenital microgastria with esophageal stenosis and diaphragmatic hernia in a 10-week old female infant. There was a small, tubular, sagittal stomach 2 × 4 cm in size with asplenia and a massively dilated intraabdominal esophagus. The gastroesophageal junction was stenotic with a firm to hard consistency. There was also a large left posterolateral congenital diaphragmatic hernia. The mega esophagus was due to distal CES. Microgastria and diaphragmatic hernia has been reported before. One case with microgastria was intrathoracic together with a small right sided diaphragmatic hernia [22].

We also report a case of thoracic stomach, congenital heart disease (large ASD and PDA), left lung hypoplasia in a case of CES. Thoracic stomach was operated in the neonatal period due to recurrent desaturations and intolerance to feeds. The diagnosis was confirmed by upper gastrointestinal study. The stenosis of the esophagus was initially missed. The patient was then operated for his cardiac condition. The patient was tolerating feeds but with occasional desaturations. His parents complained that he became intolerant to feeds when solids were introduced. Repeat esophagogram showed distal esophageal stenosis sparing the GEJ which was missed in the neonatal period (Fig. 4.2). Peptic stricture was ruled out and flexible endoscopy was normal. The patient responded well to esophageal balloon dilatation and is eating all types of food at the age of 2 years.

Table 4.1 Associated anomalies with our 27 cases of CES

Item	Number
Gastrointestinal	
EA	16 (59.3%)
Anorectal malformation	1
Thoracic stomach	1
Neurological	
Cerebral palsy/brain atrophy	4
Cardiac	
ASD	2
VSD	3
PDA	1
Skeletal	1
Others	
Down syndrome	2
Fanconi anemia	1

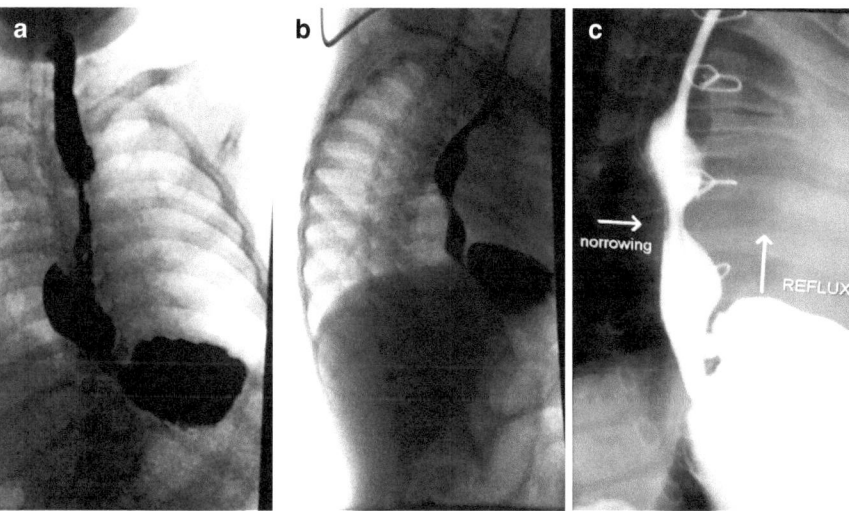

Fig. 4.2 A 2-month old boy who presented with recurrent chest problems. (**a**) Barium swallow showing partial thoracic stomach which was repaired together with Thal fundoplication. The patient was operated for PDS and VSD few months later. (**b, c**) The patient came at 18 months of age with dysphagia to semisolids. Barium swallow and meal showed a missed lower esophageal CES and mild GER. He responded well to dilatation

Incidence of CES

The true incidence of CES is not known. There are many reasons for this fact. CES can be an isolated lesion or associated with other diseases mainly esophageal atresia and/or tracheoesophageal fistula (EA and/or TEF). The isolated lesion can affect any part of the esophagus proximal to the GEJ. Also, it may involve the GEJ and behave like cardiac achalasia with diagnostic challenges. Many cases of CES affecting the GEJ are wrongly diagnosed as achalasia in infants and children. If the CES is a TBR subtype, it will not respond to dilatation or even Heller's myotomy. A resection and primary anastomosis will be required and the diagnosis is confirmed by histology [4, 11, 22]. If the CES is a FMD subtype the condition may respond to dilatation and a histological diagnosis is never obtained and the true incidence of CES is never known.

The association of CES and EA and/or TEF ranges from 0.4% to 14% [1, 2, 6]. The reason of this variation is due to difficulties in the diagnosis. The difficulties in the neonatal period are due to absence of histology specimens or failure to have a high index of suspicion during the initial esophagogram. The lesion can be at the anastomotic site of EA or distal to it. FMD responds better to dilatation, whereas the TBR usually needs resection. CES needs to be differentiated by means of histological examination at the anastomotic site or using miniprobe endoscopic ultrasonography. The presentation can be early or late. Some may have a benign course whereas others may have a very stormy one that may end up

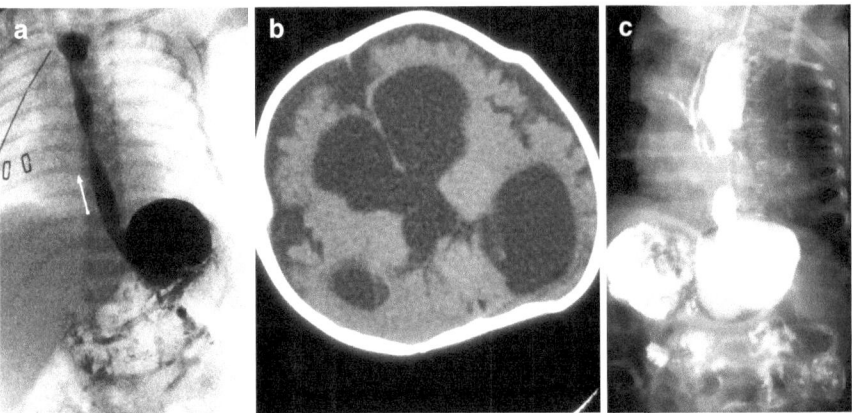

Fig. 4.3 A quadruplet (34 gestational age) operated on the 2nd day for EA/TEF. (**a**) Initial esophagogram on the 7th post operative day showed a highly suspicious narrowing in the lower esophagus proximal to the GEJ and GER. (**b**) The patient had massive aspiration requiring jet ventilation despite anti reflux measures which resulted in massive brain damage. (**c**) Repeat esophagogram confirmed the diagnosis of distal CES with recurrent TEF

with morbidity or mortality early in life [3]. For those who have a benign course, the diagnosis may be missed till the adult age. It is possible that neonatal CES are not diagnosed in the neonatal period and morbidities are attributed to associated complications like recurrent TEF or anastomotic leak (Fig. 4.3a–c). In fact these complications might be due to distal CES causing distal obstruction. Again the diagnosis of CES is missed. Recurrent TEF and anastomotic complications after EA repair (leakage or anastomotic stricture) may be a shadow for CES due to early postoperative distal obstruction [3, 6]. Dilatation is usually the initial management which may be successful and again a histological diagnosis is never obtained. For all of the above mentioned reasons the true incidence of CES is difficult to assign.

The diagnosis of CES should be considered in the neonatal period. We suggest taking samples during primary repair of EA routinely from the tips of the upper and lower pouches for histological diagnosis. A size 8 transanastomotic nasogastric tube passage during primary repair should always be practiced to diagnose a concomitant CES. However, the passage of the tube during primary repair does not rule out CES. A high index of suspicion is required during the initial esophagogram after EA repair. If there is doubt, a repeat esophagogram is encouraged.

Bluestone et al. [23] treated 24 cases of CES and almost 200 cases of EA in a single institution during the same 15-year period. The incidence of CES was estimated to be 1/25,000 live births. Fékété et al. [5] found 20 cases of CES and 484 cases of EA in the single institution during the same 25 years (1960–1984). So, the incidence of CES was lower than 1/20 of that of EA. Therefore, 1/25,000–50,000 live births is thought to be the incident rate of CES. Suzuhigashi et al. [10] published a multicenter study of 40 consecutive cases of CES in Kyushu area in Japan. They showed that the incidence of CES was 1 in every 33,000 live births. The incidence rate of EA in CES was 8/40 (20.0%). During the same period 198 patients were treated for EA from the same institutes. The incidence of CES in EA patients was 8/198 (4.0%).

In their systematic review of the English-language literature, they identified 570 studies of which 144 studies satisfied the selection criteria. The only inclusion criterion was diagnosis of CES defined as intrinsic stenosis of the esophagus. Out of three observational studies, overall frequency of FMD, TBR and MD were 53.8%, 29.9% and 16.2% respectively. Location of the stenosis in each category was assessed by using 52 reports including 64 patients. Locations were FMD mainly in the middle or lower third, TBR mainly in the lower third and MD mainly in the in the upper or middle third, as cited by Turi et al. [7].

According to 4 observational studies reviewed by Turi et al. [7] they reported an incidence rate of CES among patients with EA and/or TEF to be 9.6% (55/571). CES were located in the middle to lower third of the esophagus; 13.5% in the middle third of the esophagus and 86.5% in the lower third of the esophagus. Only in 15 cases (27% of CES cases), pathological assessment was available, 10 cases (67%) had TBR and 5 cases (33%) had FMD. The authors reported that CES in EA is not rare and warned that careful attention is required during the management of EA/TEF especially in postoperative esophagogram. According to 10 observational studies, the overall incidence rate of EA and/or TEF among patients with CES was 24.8%. The type of EA in these cases was EA in 2.4%, EA/TEF in 92.7% and TEF in 4.9% [7]

McCann [18] reported 17 cases of CES associated with EA. The overall incidence of CES with EA was 3.6%. There were 13 boys and 4 girls. Fifteen patients (88%) had a type C EA, one (6%) had a type A EA and one (6%) had an isolated TEF. Seven patients (41%) had associated anomalies (trisomy 21 in 2, VSD in 2 and VACTERL syndrome in 4).

In summary both pathologies should be discussed together. CES has been frequently associated with EA and/or TEF. Patients with severe degree of CES may die in the neonatal period undiagnosed. So, the real incidence of CES is not known. Again, this is also true because many cases will respond to dilatation alone without surgical resection losing the histological diagnosis and the exact incidence of each type of CES. Cases with isolated CES involving the GEJ, especially in neonates, infants and young children may be wrongly diagnosed as cardiac achalasia and treated as such. If dilatation is successful, the real diagnosis of FMD CES is never reached and the true incidence is again not known.

References

1. Ibrahim AHM, Al Malki TA. Congenital esophageal stenosis associated with esophageal atresia. In: Till H, Thomson M, Foker J, Holcomb G, Khan K, editors. Esophageal and gastric disorders in infancy and childhood. Berlin: Springer; 2017. p. 113–23.
2. Al Shraim MM, Ibrahim AHM, Al Malki TA, Morad N. Histopathologic profile of esophageal atresia and tracheoesophageal fistula. Ann Pediatr Surg. 2014;10:1–6.

3. Ibrahim AHM, Bazeed MF, Jamil S, Hamad HA, Abdel Raheem IM, Ashraf I. Management of congenital esophageal stenosis associated with esophageal atresia and its impact on postoperative esophageal stricture. Ann Pediatr Surg. 2016;12:36–4.

4. Al Malki TA, Ibrahim AHM. Isolated congenital esophageal stenosis: a case report and review of the literature. Ann Saudi Med. 2000;20:53–4.

5. Fékété CN, Backer AD, Jacob SL. Congenital esophageal stenosis, a review of 20 cases. Pediatr Surg Int. 1987;2:86–92.

6. Kawahara H, Imura K, Yagi M, Kubota A. Clinical characteristic of congenital oesophageal stenosis distal to associated oesophageal atresia. Surgery. 2001;129:29–3.

7. Teuri K, Saito T, Mitsunaga T, Nakata M, Yoshida H. Endoscopic management for congenital esophageal stenosis: a systematic review. World J Gastrointest Endosc. 2015;7(3):183–91.

8. Dutta HK, Mathur M, Bhatnagar V. A histopathological study of esophageal atresia and tracheoesophageal fistula. J Pediatr Surg. 2000;35:438–41.

9. Yeung CK, Spitz L, Brereton RJ, Kiely EM, Leake J, et al. Congenital esophageal stenosis due to tracheobronchial remnants: a rare but important association with esophageal atresia. J Pediatr Surg. 1992;27:852–5.

10. Suzuhigashi M, Kaji T, Nogushi H, Muto M, Goto M, Mukai M, et al. Current characteristics and management of congenital esophageal stenosis: 40 consecutive cases from a multicenter study in the Kyushu area of Japan. Pediatr Surg Int. 2017;33:1035–40.

11. El Halaby EA, El Barbary MM, Hashish AA, Kaddah SN, Hamza AF. Congenital esophageal stenosis: to dilate or to resect. Ann Pediatr Surg. 2006;2(1):2–9.

12. Yoo HJ, Kim WS, Cheon JE, Yoo SY, Park KW, Junq SE, Jung SE, et al. Congenital esophageal stenosis associated with esophageal atresia/tracheoesophageal fistula: clinical and radiologic features. Pediatr Radiol. 2010;40:1353–13590.

13. Kurian JJ, Jehangir S, Varghese IT, Thomas RJ, Mathai J, Karl S. Clinical profile and management options of children with congenital esophageal stenosis: a single center experience. J Indian Assoc Pediatr Surg. 2016;21(3):106–9.

14. Harrison CA, Katon RM. Familial multiple congenital esophageal rings: report of an affected father and son. Am J Gastroenterol. 1992;87:1813–5.

15. Rangel R, Lizarzabel M. Familial multiple congenital esophageal rings. Dig Dis. 1998;16:325.

16. Oh CH, Levine MS, Katzka DA, Rubesin SE, Pinheiro LW, Mickael A, et al. Congenital esophageal stenosis in adults: clinical and radiographic findings in seven patients. AJR. 2001;176:1179–82.

17. Coran AG, Adzick NS, Krummel TM, et al. Pediatric surgery. In: Harmon CM, Coran AG, editors. congenital anomalies of the esophagus. 7th ed. Philadelphia, PA: Elsevier; 2012. p. 893–918.

18. McCann F, Michaud L, Aspirot A, Levesque D, Gottrand F, Faure E. Congenital esophageal stenosis associated with esophageal atresia. Dis Esophagus. 2015;28:211–5.

19. Spitz L. Esophageal atresia associations. In: Till H, Thomson M, Foker J, Holocomb G, Khan KE, editors. Esophageal and gastric disorders in infancy and childhood. 1st ed. Berlin: Springer; 2017. p. 107–11.

20. Vasudevan SA, Kerendi F, Lee H, Ricketts R. Management of congenital esophageal stenosis. J Pediatr Surg. 2002;37:1024–6.

21. Sharma SC, Menon P. Congenital microgastria with esophageal stenosis and diaphragmatic hernia. Pediatr Surg Int. 2005;21:292–4.

22. Jain V, Yadav DK, Sharma S, Jana M, Gupta DK. Management of long segment congenital esophageal stenosis: a novel technique. J Indian Assoc Pediatr Surg. 2016;21:150–2.

23. Bluestone CD, Kerry R, Sieber WK. Congenital esophageal stenosis. Laryngoscope. 1969;79:1095–101.

Chapter 5
Diagnosis of CES

Diagnosis of CES

The severity of symptoms of CES is variable. The diagnosis could be difficult and tends to be delayed [1]. Symptoms of CES may begin acutely in the neonatal period with respiratory distress, pneumonia and apnea. This was reported following EA repair [2]. The clinical picture may be aggravated with a recurrent TEF or anastomotic leak due to distal esophageal obstruction [3]. This may end up with brain damage. If CES is missed during the initial esophagogram, possible complications like leakage, recurrent TEF, respiratory problems, intolerance to feeds and failure to thrive should draw our attention to look for CES during a repeat of an esophagogram. Having a high index of suspicion during the initial esophagogram is of paramount importance after EA repair to diagnose distal CES. Also, Failure to pass a size 8 French nasogastric tube to the stomach may clinch the diagnosis of CES during primary repair. However, passage of the tube to the stomach does not rule out CES [4]. Furthermore, histology obtained from biopsy specimens from the tips of the lower and/or upper pouches is also diagnostic in the neonatal period. In such later condition, the scenario of anastomotic stricture and/or major dysmotility, recurrent TEF or anastomotic leak should be anticipated. Careful handling of such cases by a nasogastric tube pump feeding and full antireflux measures should be practiced [2]. The diagnosis of CES during primary repair of EA is possible; however, simultaneous repair of the stenosis by doing a double esophageal anastomosis is a controversial approach [5]. An esophagogram demonstrating a narrow segment above the cardia is radiologically diagnostic for CES when found in the neonatal period [4, 6, 7]. In fact, this requires a high index of suspicion especially in the initial esophagogram which might be passed as normal.

However, many of the cases have delayed onset of symptoms in the form of vomiting and progressive dysphagia after the introduction of semisolid or solid food around the age of 3–6 months. A foreign body impaction in the esophagus may be the first symptom [4, 8]. Esophagogram is diagnostic by showing abrupt

© Springer Nature Switzerland AG 2019
A. Ibrahim, T. Al-Malki, *Congenital Esophageal Stenosis*,
https://doi.org/10.1007/978-3-030-10782-6_5

or tapered esophageal stenosis. This can be misdiagnosed as peptic stricture due to GER. If there is proximal esophageal dilatation the condition can be interpreted as cardiac achalasia [4]. Other modalities of investigations can help to differentiate CES, peptic stricture or cardiac achalasia from each other. These investigations include studies for GER, upper flexible esophagoscopy, esophageal manometry and EUS [9]. In CES the esophagogram will localize the stenosis and its length. There will be tertiary esophageal contractions in contrast to the aperistaltic esophageal body with failure of relaxation of the LES in cases of achalasia. At endoscopy, narrowing will have a normal appearing mucosa in contrast with the inflamed mucosa in peptic stricture and according to the type and severity of CES, the scope may or may not pass the stenotic area. Miniprobe EUS [10] is helpful in diagnosing CES and its subtype. Cardiac achalasia can be excluded by finding a normal mucosa at endoscopy, easy passage of the scope through the narrowed area. Manometry is the gold standard method of diagnosis of cardiac achalasia.

A high index of suspicion should be raised in all cases of EA. CES is an intrinsic stenosis that may be present at birth but not necessarily symptomatic [11]. Minor esophageal dysmotility as detected by barium is defined as aperistalsis, antiperistalsis, and simultaneous or uncoordinated contractions. The dysmotility is considered major if the transit time for the bolus to go to the stomach is greater than five minutes [12]. The problem of major dysmotility is that it may develop late; amenable to major complications or it can be fatal without reaching to the diagnosis of CES.

McCann et al. [13] reported 17 cases of CES associated with EA. One case was diagnosed during primary repair of EA due to inability to pass an 8 Fr tube to the stomach. In 12 patients (71%) CES was suspected by abnormal esophagogram. In seven (41%) of them, CES was diagnosed on the initial esophagogram. In five (30%), the diagnosis of CES was delayed and was diagnosed on the second or third esophagogram. The retrospective review of the previous esophagograms showed clearly the CES indicating a misinterpretation and a low index of suspicion for the diagnosis of an associated CES. Diagnosis of the remaining 4 (23%) was not possible by esophagogram but was made by esophagoscopy. In that study, all the cases of CES were localized distal to the anastomosis.

Taking a surgical specimen routinely from the tip of the esophageal pouches during primary repair of EA may show histological picture consistent with FMD or TBR [2, 12, 14]. This mandates close observation. One case in our series, the histology showed TBR with cartilage. The initial esophagogram was normal. A repeat fluoroscopic esophagogram one month later showed major esophageal dysmotility. The histologic picture confirmed the site and type of CES (Fig. 3.1a–c) [2].

Another case in our study in 2016 [2], showed distal CES and GER in the initial esophagogram after primary repair of EA/TEF at age of 10 days (Fig. 4.3a–c). Nasogastric tube feeding was started with anti reflux formula and head up position. The patient had massive aspiration and required high frequency ventilation. Repeated contrast study after weaning from ventilation showed GER, recurrent TEF and confirmed CES distal to the anastomotic site. Computed tomography of the brain showed severe brain insult.

A third example of our series is a case of a distal CES discovered during primary repair due to failure of passage of size 6 nasogastric tube. A size 5 umbilical catheter could be passed simultaneously with anterior myectomy of the distal esophagus. Histopathology showed FMD (Figs. 5.1a, b, 5.2, and 5.3). Early diagnosis of CES with EA/TEF can be made by taking histology specimens from the tips of the esophageal pouches during primary repair or failure to pass a size 8 nasogastric tube distally. A high index of suspicion is required during the initial esophagogram to diagnose distal CES. CES distal to the anastomotic site is suspected by a segmental, smooth, circumferential narrowing in the distal esophagus 2–6 cm above the GEJ. It is easy to miss it and pass it as a normal peristaltic wave or an impression [6]. Errors in the diagnosis at the initial esophagogram and omitting taking histological samples during primary repair make the true incidence difficult to assess and may lead to morbidity and even mortality without knowing the exact etiology [2].

The late onset diagnosis of CES is suspected by the clinical triad of recurrent aspiration, dysphagia and FTT together with the aid of an esophagogram. Patients may present with distal esophageal foreign bodies [4]. Improvement of the feeding process with the insertion of a feeding nasogastric tube is diagnostic of a problem

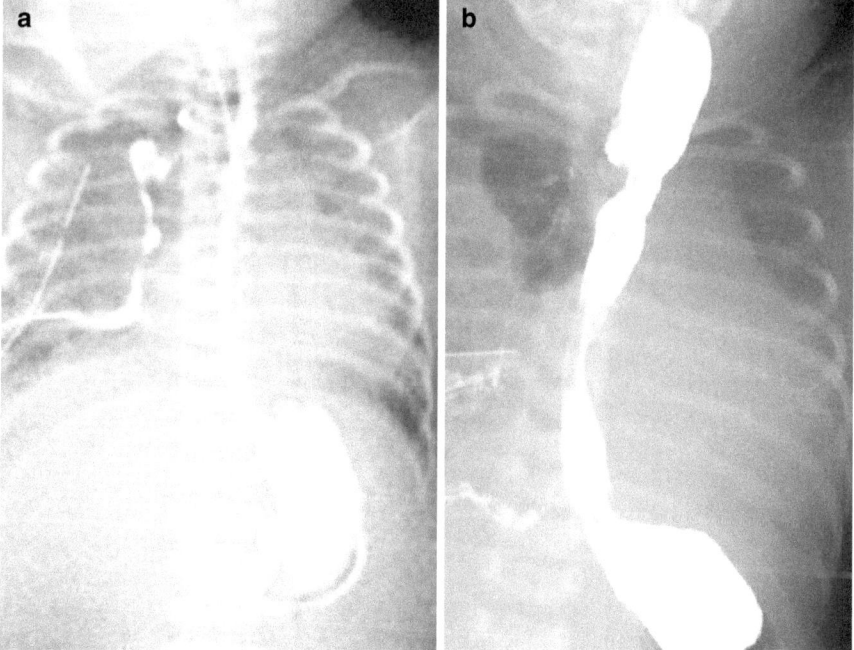

Fig. 5.1 A 34-week gestational age newborn operated for EA, discovered to have a distal CES due to failure to pass a size 6 NGT during primary repair. Myectomy was done with passage of a size 5 umbilical catheter to the stomach. (**a**) Initial esophagogram showed anastomotic leak. (**b**) Repeat esophagogram confirmed a distal CES with resolution of the anastomotic leak

Fig. 5.2 The previous case after complete resolution of leakage; three sessions of esophageal dilatation together with lower esophageal myectomy, Thal fundoplication and gastrostomy were successful to start oral feeding within 2 months

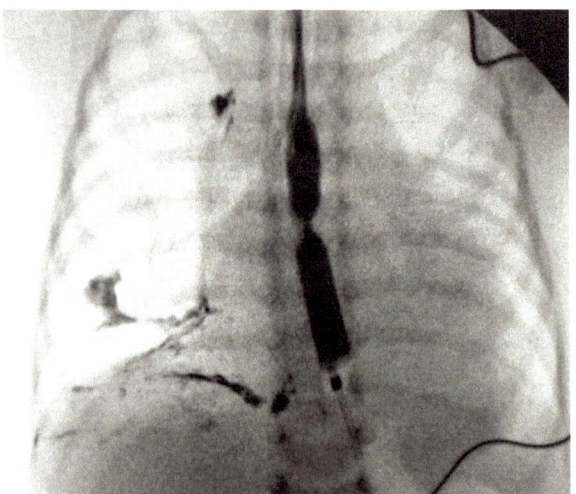

Fig. 5.3 Histology of the myectomy specimen of the previous case showing FMD

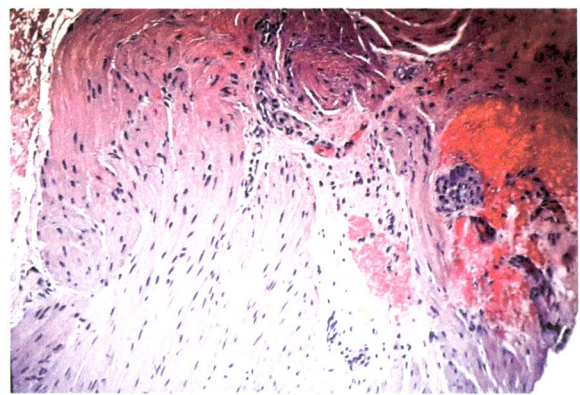

in the esophagus itself. A barium study is the diagnostic and follow-up tool. Full cooperation and mutual understanding of the pathology between the radiologist and the surgeon is required.

GER in cases of EA with CES is said to be unlikely to be present [15]. This is true when the CES involves the GEJ behaving like achalasia. However, we believe, like others, that it is common [2, 3, 12, 16]. Monitoring of pH, esophagoscopy with biopsy, and possibly manometry may be required [17]. Despite all of these investigations, it may be difficult to differentiate between CES and stricture caused by GER [4]. Diagnostic Errors are common since most of these patients are diagnosed and treated as peptic stricture [4, 16].

It is important to precisely diagnose CES preoperatively. The type of stricture will determine the modality of treatment [18]. It is difficult to differentiate between FMD and TBR without the preliminary histologic picture, or miniprobe EUS, preoperatively. A correct preoperative diagnosis of the underlying etiology of stenosis was not reached in most cases in a review of the literature for 59 cases with TBR with cartilage. The majority were diagnosed as peptic stricture or achalasia [19]. Esophagoscopy with biopsy may fail to diagnose deep seated ectopic tissue [11, 20]. Abrupt narrowing as seen fluoroscopically may be seen in cases of TBR while narrowing of the FMD may show more gradual, regular and well centered appearance. However these typical findings with fluoroscopy are not always present [18]. The presence of a short, sharp waist like impression which suddenly disappears with increased pressure during balloon dilatation, means the presence of cartilaginous rings [4]. CT scan and MRI as well as conventional imaging tools cannot differentiate TBR from FMD [9]. However, miniprobe endoscopic ultrasonography (EUS) is said to be helpful to differentiate TBR with cartilage from FMD [9, 10, 21]. The success rate of dilatation for CES with EUS was 90% and it was 29% without it. The rate of perforation with or without EUS case selection was 7% and 24%, respectively [22]. Hence, there was a high success rate for dilatation with low rate of perforation with case selection using EUS.

Intra operative palpation and the use of the flexible Esophagoscopy may be of help [18]. The authors found that intra operative palpation of the lesion is not always easy. However, these modalities suspect but do not confirm the presence and the type of CES. The diagnosis is only confirmed by the histologic picture. If palpation is doubtful, then, it is advisable to proceed for a frozen section biopsy. The results are available within 15–30 min and are accurate in comparison to cases of Hirschsprung's disease frozen section biopsy which are lengthy, sometimes inaccurate and requires expert pediatric histopathologists.

The diagnosis of CES associated with EA is difficult and treatment is usually delayed [13]. A high index of suspicion for associated CES is required especially in the presence of post-operative complications like dysphagia, recurrent TEF, leakage, anastomotic stricture, food impaction, feeding difficulties, FTT and respiratory symptoms [23]. More than one esophagogram may be, required, because the diagnosis of CES may be missed or misinterpreted as transient spasm, dysmotility, or esophageal narrowing due to reflux [6]. Endoscopy suspects the diagnosis of CES by revealing normal esophageal mucosa and esophageal narrowing distal to the anastomosis.

Upper Gastrointestinal Contrast Studies (UGI)

This is a radiographic contrast study of the esophagus, stomach and duodenum. It is simple, quickly performed, with a low radiation dose, inexpensive, and does not need sedation. It gives important and useful anatomical, morphological, and functional data. The child's clinical status including history should be obtained before the study. It is the primary imaging technique in patients with history of dysphagia, intolerance to feed and aspiration. This clinical condition is due to a wide range of abnormalities, all of which should be searched for during the study. Hence, a special attention is required.

Normal Anatomy and Physiology of the Esophagus

The esophagus starts at the level of the cricopharyngeus muscle (upper esophageal sphincter or UES) to the GEJ (lower esophageal sphincter or LES). The normal esophageal extrinsic impressions are the cricopharyngeal muscle, aortic impression, left main bronchus, left atrium and the diaphragm [24]. The anatomy in neonates and infants is different than in adults. Mouth and pharynx are close together, the larynx is higher and smaller. Coordination of swallowing is not usually present before 36 weeks of gestation. There is a higher incidence of GER in infants and neonates due to a less acute angle of His and a shorter intra-abdominal portion of the esophagus [24].

Technique of UGI Study

To reduce the dose of radiation, a digital pulsed fluoroscopy and video fluoroscopy is used. A special equipment is adapted for neonates and infants for better immobilization, proper position and limitation of field view. The contrast of choice is barium sulfate unless the patient is a neonate with suspected TEF, esophageal perforation, or aspiration. Hence, a low osmolar nonionic iodine contrast material (Iopamidol 61.24%w/v) is preferred to decrease the risk of cardiovascular compromise [25]. A team work is mandatory in our institution which is composed of a pediatric surgeon and a radiologist following the three phase's protocol. Using the bottle, the first oral phase of swallowing is assessed. In the second pharyngeal phase, the hypo pharynx elevates, the epiglottis deflects, pharynx contracts and the cricopharyngeus muscle relax. The third esophageal phase starts from the UES to the LES. Actually, a complete UGI series is performed rather than an esophagogram [25].

We start the study by using the bottle to evaluate the oral and pharyngeal phase of swallowing. We then use an NGT in the mid esophagus starting in the semi prone position to evaluate for TEF then supine to continue evaluating the esophageal phase.

Evaluating the Oral and Pharyngeal Phase

In cerebral palsy, there are difficulties in sucking, chewing and voluntary movements of the mouth (cortical motor deficits). Pharyngeal phase dysfunction occurs with brain stem lesions. Combined oropharyngeal dysfunction occurs in diffuse hypoxic—ischemic injury [26]. Nasopharyngeal reflux is the most common pathology in this area due to failure of soft palate elevation mechanism leading to aspiration in neonates and infants. This can be treated simply by changing feed consistency. Cricopharyngeal dysfunction should be differentiated from the normal asymptomatic cricopharyngeal impression.

Esophageal Phase Evaluation

Oropharyngeal disorders, Laryngeal clefts, cricopharyngeal spasm or achalasia can lead to life threatening pulmonary aspiration. This is also possible in many other esophageal lesions like, motility disorders, TEF, CES including vascular rings, cardiac achalasia, hiatus hernia and GER. If in doubt, a low osmolar non iodine contrast material (Iopamidol) should be used with suction devices available [26].

Esophageal motility disorders are evaluated using real-time fluoroscopy. There are three types of peristaltic waves. The primary peristaltic wave is initiated by a bolus and is a progressing distally with lumen diminishing contraction wave propelling the bolus through the esophagus. The secondary peristaltic wave follows the primary to clear all the remaining contrast material from the esophagus. The tertiary waves are pathologic non propulsive, uncoordinated contractions not seen in healthy children. Antiperistaltic waves in the lower esophagus are nonspecific and can be seen in GER, motility disorders, and after surgery. The risk of aspiration is very high in aperistalsis due to neuromuscular disorder. LES disorders like achalasia, isolated CES and GER are important dysfunction that needs to be studied and evaluated [26].

Esophagogram, bronchoscopy and esophagoscopy are required for the diagnosis of isolated TEF together with fistula stenting (Fig. 5.4a, b). The pull-back tube esophagogram technique is useful. The fistula is not actually an H-type but N-type with the transverse limb coming upwards from the esophagus to the trachea which is anterior to the esophagus. The fistula will not be seen during normal swallowing.

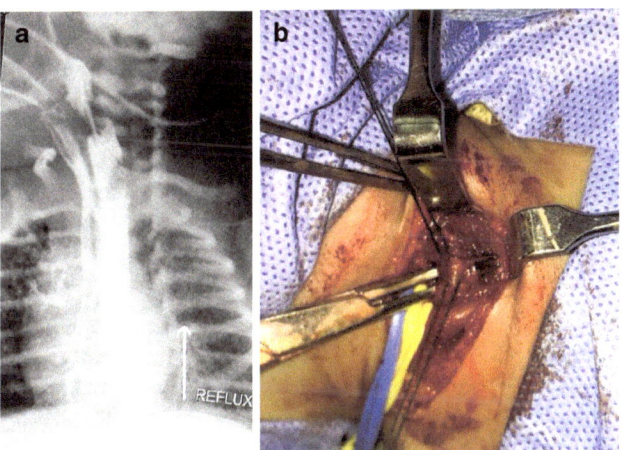

Fig. 5.4 (**a**) An esophagogram (using the feeding tube pull-up technique in the semi prone position) showing the N-type fistula. Upward reflux of the water soluble contrast material into the esophagus will show the fistula clearly. (**b**) Confirmation of the fistula and its location by tracheoscopy and fistula stenting is followed by exploration. In this case a cervical approach with full neck extension is used to ligate the fistula. The blue sling is used for the carotid artery, the yellow for the esophagus and the black stay sutures for the fistula

It might be seen if the patient is semi prone with the NGT in the lower, mid and upper esophagus with injection of the contrast distending the esophagus from down-upwards [25].

CES associated with EA can affect the esophagus at the anastomotic area in EA. Esophagogram may show severe stricture at the anastomotic site or major esophageal dysmotility [2, 12]. Also, it can be distal to the anastomotic site sparing the GEJ. The triad of stricture, dysmotility and GER is common. The isolated type of CES usually affects the distal esophagus sparing GEJ with the same possible triad of stricture, dysmotility and GER. If it involves the GEJ, then it will behave like cardiac achalasia. Esophagogram will show a bird beak like appearance and the proximal dilated esophagus showing tertiary peristaltic non propulsive waves [27]. In cardiac achalasia, esophagogram shows normal swallowing with normal peristalsis to the level of aortic arch. Early in the course, uncoordinated peristalsis is found in the distal esophagus and the pathognomonic sign of lower esophageal peaking is seen. In the advanced state, the proximal dilated esophagus usually will be aperistaltic [28]. Manometry or combined videomanometry will be of great help to differentiate CES from achalasia [29].

The isolated distal CES or that associated with EA is very difficult to be diagnosed in the initial esophagogram unless there is a very high index of suspicion. The pathology can be passed as normal (a peristaltic wave or an impression). This is because CES can be asymptomatic early in life and symptoms are delayed for some unknown period of time. The symptoms once develop can be very severe to endanger life or mild to be tolerated for a long period of time. Because of this, nobody knows how many patients are undiagnosed and what the real incidence of CES is.

CES should be differentiated from acquired esophageal stenosis due to GER, Candida albicans, herpes simplex virus, epidermolysis bullosa dystrophica, cytomegalovirus, caustic ingestion, graft versus- host disease, Crohn's granulomatous disease, and radiation therapy. Acquired stenosis can also be due to trauma, iatrogenic surgical or endoscopic treatment. For eosinophilic esophagitis endoscopy and biopsy are required for diagnosis. During esophagogram, the exact location, length and diameter of the stenosis and the presence of prestenotic dilatation, the rigidity of the stenosis and the presence of an associated membranous web should be determined [25].

Disorders of GEJ

The common disorders of the GEJ are; sliding hiatal hernia with or without GER, paraesophageal hernia, achalasia and CES. Disorders of GEJ are common after repair EA. The disorders of the GEJ include GER, hiatal hernia, achalasia and Isolated CES involving the GEJ. In a paraesophageal hernia, the GEJ remains in the abdomen and may be complicated with gastric volvulus and obstruction. However, in sliding hiatal hernia, the GEJ is in the thorax encouraging GER. A pathologic GER is diagnosed if there is lack of response to dietary and postural antireflux measure. If there is Failure to thrive, acute respiratory events, chronic respiratory symptoms, and / or bronchospasm contrast swallow and meal are indicated [30]. The study will show anatomic and physiologic abnormalities. It will show any site of obstruction, aspiration, and complications of GER like esophagitis, dysmotility, ulcerations, and strictures. Also it will rule out malrotation, pyloric or duodenal obstruction [25].

Anatomical and Functional Causes for GER in EA/TEF Patients

EA itself and the anatomic changes due to its repair compromise the delicate antireflux mechanisms [26, 31]. The GEJ may be congenitally abnormal with a shorter intrabdominal esophagus and a larger hiatus inviting a sliding hernia and GER. Anastomotic tension plays a major role in inducing GER. The clearing of the refluxate by esophageal peristaltic pump is also damaged as proved by contrast studies, Manometry, and combined pH-metering and impedance studies. There is distal esophageal aperistalsis with poor progressive weak waves through the entire esophagus. Dysmotility can be due to the marked disproportion between the upper pouch and the fistulous pouch. There is muscle distortion by glands, fibrosis and associated CES [2, 12, 14]. Damage to the extrinsic and intrinsic innervations and abnormal distributions of the neuronal structures are also abnormal as mentioned in the chapter of motility disorder. Extra esophageal reasons include Gastrostomy, tracheomalacia, abnormal gastric motility and gastric emptying.

Outside Impressions of the Esophagus

Esophageal impressions may be normal physiological or pathological. Normal esophageal impressions were discussed before. Pathological impressions include vascular rings and less commonly compression by mediastinal masses. Vascular rings are known causes of CES due to outside compression of the esophagus but they are not included in the definition of CES proposed by Fékété. Whether they should be included in the classification of CES is a matter of discussion. However the vascular rings should be considered in the etiology of CES because the condition is congenital stenosis of the esophagus.

Double Aortic Arch

A double aortic arch is the most common vascular ring causing congenital pathological outside impression of the esophagus [32]. It is caused by failure of regression of the right aortic arch which normally gets absorbed between the right subclavian artery and its junction with the descending aorta. The remnant of the right arch will form the right innominate artery. Failure of this process of absorption in the right arch produces a vascular ring and the esophagus and trachea are completely encircled and compressed leading to, stridor, respiratory distress and dysphagia. The condition is usually an isolated lesion but is sometimes associated with septal defects, tetralogy of Fallots, or transposition of the great vessels [32]. Presenting symptoms includes stridor (100%), persistent cough (75%), chronic dyspnea (75%), reflex apnea (60%), recurrent upper respiratory tract infection (56%) and dysphagia (25%) [33].

When a vascular ring is clinically suspected an esophagogram is the first screening test [25]. A high index of suspicion is required. An anterior S-shaped indentation in the frontal projection is highly suggestive of a double aortic arch (Fig. 5.5a, b). A

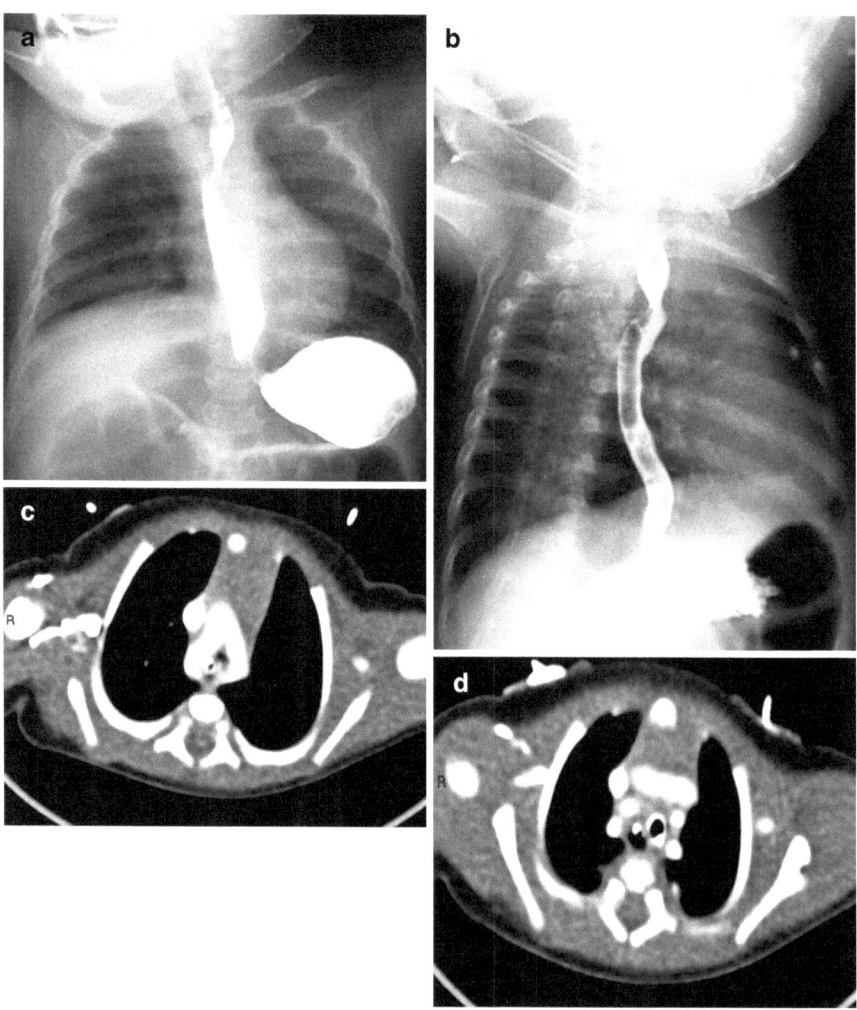

Fig. 5.5 Double aortic arch (**a**, **b**) an esophagogram showing esophageal indentation from anterior, posterior and from both sides. (**c**, **d**) CT angiogram showing that the right side is dominant

posterior indentation may or may not be a vascular ring. If a right aortic arch is present, a vascular ring is highly suspected. Some may consider flexible bronchoscopy as the first line of investigation especially for stridor in the neonate. Esophagoscopy may also be indicated for dysphagia. Spiral CT will show the lesion causing the extra mural compressing. Echocardiography is an important noninvasive technique for diagnosing vascular rings. Angiography will confirm the diagnosis (Fig. 5.5c, d). Surgical division of the non-dominant arch is effective and safe at the age of one year.

Left Sided Aortic Arch with an Aberrant Right Subclavian Artery

This is rarely present which is usually asymptomatic. However, dysphagia, cough, stridor due to compression of the esophagus or the trachea may be present (Fig. 5.6a–c).

Right Aortic Arch (RAA)

RAA is a rare anomaly where the aortic arch is on the right side of the vertebral column. It is present in 0.1% of the general population and in 1.8–3.6% in cases of EA [34]. Other associated anomalies with RAA include, septal defects (in 50% of EA cases with RAA), Fallots' tetralogy (in 20–25% of Fallots), aberrant left subclavian artery usually with patent ductus arteriosus forming a complete vascular ring [34] (Fig. 5.7a–e).

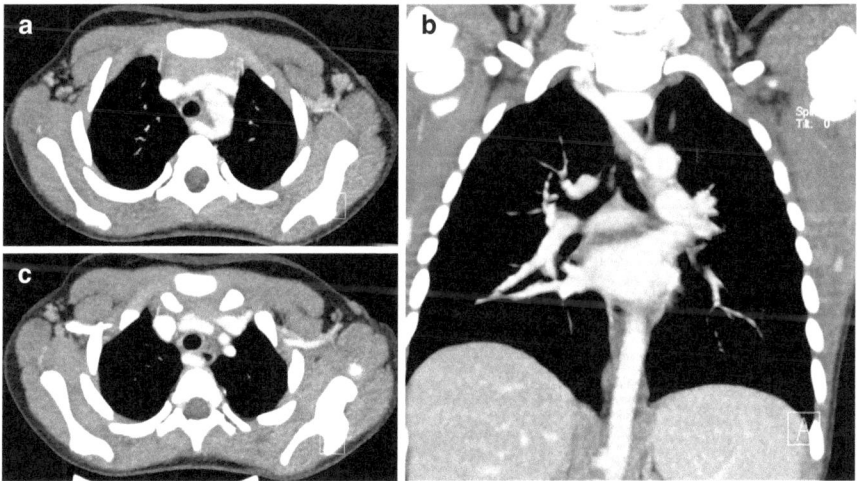

Fig. 5.6 (**a–c**) CT angiogram showing left aortic arch with aberrant right subclavian artery

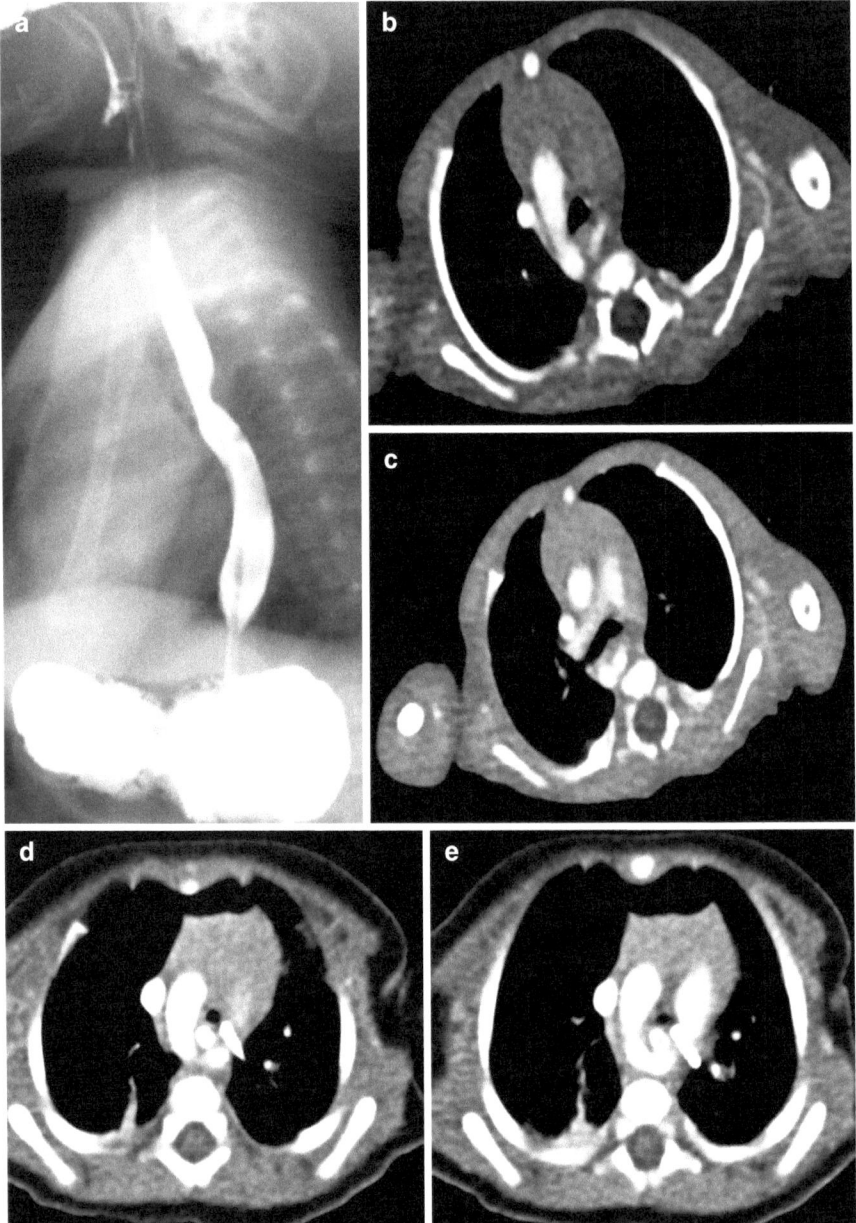

Fig. 5.7 Right aortic arch (**a**) esophagogram showing posterior smooth indentation of the esophagus. (**b**, **c**) CT angiogram showing right aortic arch with left aberrant subclavian artery. (**d**, **e**) CT
angiogram of another case of right aortic arch with aberrant left subclavian artery with clamped
aortopulmonary shunt at the level of origin of the aberrant left subclavian

If the left aortic arch disappears instead and the right arch persists, a right aortic arch develops. The aberrant subclavian artery may be seated behind the esophagus in 80%, between the esophagus and trachea in 15% and anterior to the trachea in 5% [35]. Canty et al. highlighted that when RAA is associated with EA, the gap length is long and that an infant with a long gap is 19 times as likely to have an associated RAA [36]. Three types of RAA are documented: (1) those with mirror image branching (2) those with aberrant left subclavian artery and (3) those with isolated left subclavian artery.

The isolated RAA is usually asymptomatic. That with associated aberrant left subclavian artery can be diagnosed antenatally. Complications are rare in the neonatal period. Respiratory compression and dysphagia can occur in infancy and adulthood [37]. When RAA is suspected with EA, preoperative diagnosis should be confirmed by a three dimensional echocardiogram. Preoperative tracheoscopy can help to look for the dominant pulsations in the right side, to diagnose a proximal pouch TEF and finally the gap length. During surgery, a left thoracotomy or thoracoscopic approach seems more appropriate to expose the esophagus, to close a patent ductus arteriosus and treat a vascular ring if RAA is confirmed preoperatively. However the right sided approach is valid and has no increased complication rates and no negative effects on the outcome. If a long gap is suspected preoperatively, a left approach should be a better option. If no long gap is suspected either right or left approach can be used.

If a RAA is discovered only during right thoracotomy and the dissection is easy the anastomosis can be completed. If it is difficult or long gap, the fistula can be divided as a first step and later left thoracotomy or thoracoscopic approach can be the second step after full evaluation of the vascular anomalies [34].

Pulmonary Artery Sling

A pulmonary artery sling is suspected when there is a focal nodular indentation on the anterior portion of the esophagus at the level of the carina on lateral esophagogram. A left sided aortic arch with aberrant right subclavian artery causes a posterior esophageal indentation. The pulmonary artery sling (PAS) is rare. In this anomaly, the left pulmonary artery (LPA) stems from the posterior portion of the right pulmonary artery. The LPA (frequently hypoplastic) goes to the left positioning itself between the trachea anteriorly and the esophagus posteriorly compressing both structures. This produces respiratory symptoms and feeding difficulty. The respiratory symptoms may be acutely presented with possible fatal outcome [38]. Associated cardiac defects include septal defects, patent ductus arteriosus, and persistent left superior vena cava connected to the coronary sinus. Other associated anomalies include right lung hypoplasia, tracheal stenosis and right tracheal bronchus [39]. Diagnosis is made by three-dimensional echocardiography, spiral computed tomography and MR angiography.

Surgical correction is need. The LPA is disinserted and reimplanted to the main pulmonary artery. The treatment of tracheal stenosis is debatable and will depend on the severity. If the stenosis is short, then reimplantation of LPA is enough. If the tracheal stenosis is long then the options are tracheoplasty using autologous material and slide tracheoplasty. Endoscopic techniques may also be utilized by performing dilatation or stenting with good results [39].

References

1. Kim S-H, Kim H-Y, Jung S-EU, Lee S-C, Park K-W. Clinical study of congenital esophageal stenosis: comparison according to association of esophageal atresia and tracheoesophageal fistula. Pediatr Gastroenterol Hepatol Nutr. 2017;20(2):79–86.
2. Ibrahim AHM, Bazeed MF, Jamil S, Hamad HA, Abdel Raheem IM, Ashraf I. Management of congenital esophageal stenosis associated with esophageal atresia and its impact on postoperative esophageal stricture. Ann Pediatr Surg. 2016;12:36–4.
3. Kawahara H, Imura K, Yagi M, Kubota A. Clinical characteristic of congenital oesophageal stenosis distal to associated oesophageal atresia. Surgery. 2001;129:29–3.
4. Neilson IR, Croitoru DP, Guttman FM, Yossef S, Laberge JM. Distal congenital esophageal stenosis associated with esophageal atresia. J Pediatr Surg. 1991;26:478–82.
5. Margarit J, Castanon M, Muntaner RJ, Lee KW, Salarich J. Congenital esophageal stenosis associated with tracheoesophageal fistula. Pediatr Surg Int. 1994;9:577–8.
6. Yoo HJ, Kim WS, Cheon JE, Yoo SY, Park KW, Junq SE, et al. Congenital esophageal stenosis associated with esophageal atresia/tracheoesophageal fistula: clinical and radiologic features. Pediatr Radiol. 2010;40:1353–9.
7. Raffensperger JG. Congenital esophageal stenosis. In: Swenson pediatric surgery. 5th ed. Norwalk, CT: Appleton and Lange; 1990. p. 719–20.
8. Bluestone CD, Kerry R, Sieber WK. Congenital esophageal stenosis. Laryngoscope. 1969;79:1095–101.
9. Usui N, Kamata S, Kawahara H, Sawai T, Nakajim K, Soh H, et al. Usefulness of endoscopic ultrasonography in the diagnosis of congenital esophageal stenosis. J Pediatr Surg. 2002;37:1744–6.
10. Lee KS. Preoperative diagnosis of congenital esophageal stenosis caused by tracheobronchial remnants using miniprobe endoscopic ultrasonography in a child. Pediatr Gastroenterol Hepatol Nutr. 2012;15(1):52–6.
11. Fékété CN, Backer AD, Jacob SL. Congenital esophageal stenosis, a review of 20 cases. Pediatr Surg Int. 1987;2:86–92.
12. Ibrahim AH, Al Malki TA, Hamza AF, Bahnasy AF. Congenital esophageal stenosis associated with esophageal atresia: new concepts. Pediatr Surg Int. 2007;23:533–7.
13. McCann F, Michaud L, Aspirot A, Levesque D, Gottrand F, Faure C. Congenital esophageal stenosis associated with esophageal atresia. Dis Esophagus. 2015;28:211–5.
14. Al Shraim MM, Ibrahim AHM, Al Malki TA, Morad N. Histopathologic profile of esophageal atresia and tracheoesophageal fistula. Ann Pediatr Surg. 2014;10:1–6.
15. Dominguez R, Zarabi M, Oh KS, Bender TM, Girdany BR. Congenital esophageal stenosis. Clin Radiol. 1985;36:263–6.
16. Yeung CK, Spitz L, Brereton RJ, Kiely EM, Leak J. Congenital esophageal stenosis due to tracheobronchial remnants: a rare but important association with esophageal atresia. J Pediatr Surg. 1992;27:852–5.
17. Amae S, Nio M, Kamiyama T, Ishil T, Yoshida S, Hayashi Y, et al. Clinical characteristics and management of congenital esophageal stenosis: a report on 14 cases. J Pediatr Surg. 2003;38:565–70.

18. Takamizawa S, Tsugawa C, Mouri N, Satoh S, Kaneqwa K, Nishijima E, et al. Congenital esophageal stenosis: therapeutic strategy based on etiology. J Pediatr Surg. 2002;37:197–201.
19. Zhao L-L, Hsieh W-S, Hsu W-M. Congenital esophageal stenosis owing to ectopic tracheobronchial remnants. J Pediatr Surg. 2004;39:1183–7.
20. Murphy SG, Yazbeck S, Russon P. Isolated congenital esophageal stenosis. J Pediatr Surg. 1995;30:1238–41.
21. Kouchi K, Yoshida H, Matsunage T, Ohtsuka Y, Nagatake E, Satoh Y, Terue K, Mitsunage T, et al. Endosonographic evaluation in two children with esophageal stenosis. J Pediatr Surg. 2002;37:934–6.
22. Teuri K, Saito T, Mitsunaga T, Nakata M, Yoshida H. Endoscopic management for congenital esophageal stenosis: a systematic review. World J Gastrointest Endosc. 2015;7(3):183–91.
23. Krishnan U, Moussa H, Dall' Oglio L, Homaira N, Rosen R, et al. ESPGHAN-NASPGHAN Guidelines for the evaluation and treatment of gastrointestinal and nutritional complications in children with esophageal atresia- tracheoesophageal fistula. JPGN. 2016;63(5):550–70.
24. Solvis TL. The normal esophagus. In: Solvis TL, et al., editors. Caffey's pediatric diagnostic imaging. 11th ed. Philadelphia, PA: Mosby; 2008. p. 2005–12.
25. Kljucevsek D. A pictorial essay on radiography of swallowing and esophageal disorders. Pediatr Today. 2015;11(1):10–23.
26. Solvis TL. Disorders of deglutition, peristalsis, and the velopharyngeal portal. In: Solvis TL, et al., editors. Caffey's pediatric diagnostic imaging. 11th ed. Philadelphia, PA: Mosby; 2008. p. 2021–6.
27. Al Malki TA, Ibrahim AHM. Isolated congenital esophageal stenosis: a case report and review of the literature. Ann Saudi Med. 2000;20:53–4.
28. Eckardt AJ, Eckardt VF. Current clinical approach to achalasia. World J Gastroenterol. 2009;32:3969–75.
29. Kawahara H, Kubota A, Okuyama H, Oue T, Tazuke Y, Okada A. The usefulness of videomanometry for studying pediatric esophageal motor disease. J Pediatr Surg. 2004;39:1754–7.
30. Lightdale JR, Gremse DA. Section on gastroenterology, hepatology and nutrition. Gastroesophageal reflux: management guidance for the pediatrician. Pediatrics. 2013;131(5):e1684–95.
31. Tovar JA, Fragoso AC. Gastroesophageal reflux after repair of esophageal atresia. Eur J Pediatr Surg. 2013;23:175–81.
32. Chan YT, NG DKK, Chong ASF, Ho JCS. Double aortic arch presenting as neonatal stridor. J Pediatr. 2003;8:126–9.
33. Gormley PK, Colreavy MP, Patil N, Woods AE. Congenital vascular anomalies and persistent respiratory symptoms in children. Int J Pediatr Otorhinolaryngol. 1999;51:23–31.
34. Parolini F, Armellini A, Boroni G, Bagolan P, Alberti D. The management of newborns with esophageal atresia and right aortic arch: a systematic review or still unsolved problem. J Pediatr Surg. 2016;51:304–9.
35. Arazinska A, Polguj M, Szymczyk K, Kaczmarska M, Trebinski L. Right aortic arch analysis – anatomical variant or serious vascular defect? BMC Cardiovasc Disord. 2017;17:102–8.
36. Canty JR, Boyle JREM, Linden B, Healey PJ, Tapper D, Hall DG, Sawin RS, Foker JE, et al. Aortic arch anomalies associated with long gap esophageal atresia and tracheoesophageal fistula. J Pediatr Surg. 1997;32(11):1587–91.
37. Tschirch E, Chaoui R, Wauer RR, Schnider M, Rudiger M. Perinatal management of right aortic arch with aberrant left subclavian artery associated with critical stenosis of the subclavian artery in a newborn. Ultrasound Obstet Gynecol. 2005;25:296–8.
38. Castaneda AR, Jonas RA, Mayer JRJE, Hanley FL. Vascular rings, slings and tracheal anomalies. In: Castaneda AR, Jonas RA, Mayer JRJE, Hanley FL, editors. Cardiac surgery of the neonate and infant. Philadelphia, PA: WB Saunders; 1994. p. 397–408.
39. Carretero JM, Huertas M, Prada F, Rissech M, Jimenez L, Bartrons J, et al. Surgical treatment of anomalous left pulmonary artery. Rev Esp Cardiol. 2011;64(4):338–41.

Chapter 6
Treatment of CES

There is no consensus about the treatment of CES. The two main lines of treatment include conservative dilatation or surgical resection. As we proceed with the coming pages for treating CES, we will see that dealing with CES associated with EA is much more difficult than the isolated type of CES. While the later is straight forward yet CES associated with EA is more complex and protracted. This is true despite the fact that the main lines of treatment are essentially the same; dilatation and resection. It is enough to mention that 11 patients out of 16 (68.75%) of the patients with CES associated with EA required fundoplication with gastrostomy in order to proceed with management of these patients safely. The reason is the ominous triad of stenosis, dysmotility and GER.

Dilatation of CES

Conservative management involves endoscopic or fluoroscopic guided dilatation(s) of CES with balloon or Savary dilators under general anesthesia. Dilatation is attempted as a first step treatment in all patients. Esophageal dilatation remains the main treatment for esophageal stenosis. Current evidence supports the popularity of balloons over bougies [1]. Choice of dilatation technique (bouginage or balloon dilators) depends on personal experience or preference of the operator. The advantage of hydrostatic balloon dilators is the radial force applied on the stricture while avoiding axial forces. Savory-Gilliard semi-rigid dilators apply radial force on the stricture but also an axial one with stricture stretching and greater esophageal trauma. Bougies exceptionally are better in long and tortuous stricture and severely fibrotic ones [2].The procedure should be performed in children under general anesthesia with tracheal intubation. To avoid risk of perforation, a guide wire is introduced under endoscopic or fluoroscopic control. No controlled studies have been reported to suggest a better safety for one dilator type over the other. In case of difficulty, the guide wire can be pushed to the stomach under fluoroscopic control

© Springer Nature Switzerland AG 2019
A. Ibrahim, T. Al-Malki, *Congenital Esophageal Stenosis*,
https://doi.org/10.1007/978-3-030-10782-6_6

or endoscopic guidance. The balloon can be filled with water or contrast medium. Using the contrast allows monitoring the disappearance of the waist in the balloon indicating successful dilatation of the stricture. The procedure is only partially successful if the waist persists [3]. Post dilatation x-ray or endoscopic evaluation is helpful to rule out perforation. No controlled studies to determine the optimal number of dilatations and the optimal interval between dilatation sessions. The interval can be 7 days, 15 days and 21–30 days. The interval also can be based on the severity of the stricture, symptoms of relapse or recurrence. TBR can be distinguished before dilatation by using endoscopic ultrasonography (EUS) [4–6]. Overall success rate of dilatation for CES with or without case selection by using EUS was 90% and 29%, respectively. Overall rate of perforation with or without case selection was 7% and 24%, respectively [7]. Endoscopic dilatation has been established by some authors as a primary therapy for CES except TBR subtype. Surgery is reserved for cases when dilatations have failed or in cases of TBR [8].

CES in the neonatal period should have utmost attention. Failure of early diagnosis and treatment may end up with morbidities and even mortality without diagnosis. We believe that routine histopathology for specimens from the upper and lower pouches during primary repair of EA may help early diagnosis, subtyping and treatment. A nasogastric tube size 8 should be passed through the lower pouch to the stomach. However, successful passage of the tube to the stomach does not rule out CES. A normal early fluoroscopic Barium swallow and meal does not exclude CES and must be repeated at 4–6 weeks if CES is suspected. A high index of suspicion should be practiced during the initial esophagogram. If this is suspicious, an esophageal balloon should be tried 3 weeks after primary surgery for EA. If stenosis is confirmed, EUS should be used (if the facility and experience are available) for typing and selecting cases of TBR for shorter periods of dilatation. FMD are offered longer periods for balloon dilatations. The development of the triad of esophageal dysmotility, GER, and stricture should be managed as early as possible. By doing this, the consequences of malnutrition, recurrent aspiration and even mortality can be avoided. Full antireflux measures and balloon dilatation for stricture should be initiated. If the dysmotility is major, a partial anterior wrap together with a feeding gastrostomy are indicated. During the procedure, a myectomy as long as possible of the lengthened lower esophagus is taken and sent for histopathologic and possibly histochemical examination [3].

For those cases discovered late, proper chest treatment, antireflux measures and nutritional support should be started. Nasogastric tube feeding is very useful. If GER develops, antireflux measures or even pump feeding should be tried. Antireflux measures together with balloon dilatation should be the initial treatment of all forms of CES [8, 9].

Most cases with TBR without cartilage respond well to medical antireflux measures. Three out of four required a single balloon dilatation and the fourth one did not require dilatation. The four patients showed excellent long term clinical outcome despite of persistence of radiological minor dysmotility.

Surgery for CES

Cases with TBR with cartilage may require a limited surgical resection and primary anastomosis if balloon dilatations fails with three to five sessions according to the response [4–6]. Surgical resection will also be indicated if initial sufficient dilatation is not achieved or symptoms recur very soon after dilatation [13]. Some authors experienced severe complications with repeated dilatations in CES [4, 10, 11, 14]. The role played by adjuncts to dilatation and stents will be discussed separately.

The extent of TBR into the distal esophagus should be accurately assessed during surgery. If palpation of the distal esophagus is suspicious, frozen section biopsy is required. A fundoplication is recommended after resection if it disturbs the gastro esophageal junction to avoid the possible post-operative complications of GER and hiatus hernia [3, 12, 14–16]. Circular myectomy was performed successfully for the treatment of CES due to TBR [17, 18]. Thoracoscopic resection of a distal CES and esophageal end to end anastomosis was successfully performed [19]. A laparoscopic lower esophageal stricturoplasty with anterior fundoplication for CES due to TBR was also successful [20]. Surgical resection may be complicated by recurrent stricture that may require repeated post-operative dilatations.

Cases with FMD usually respond better to balloon dilatations [3, 9, 10]. However, a limited surgical resection may be required even for FMD if dilatations fail [10, 12, 21].

The incidence of anastomotic stricture after repair of EA ranges from 18 to 50% [22, 23]. The etiology of such stricture is not known. Risk factors include anastomotic leakage, tension at the anastomotic site, a two-layer anastomosis and gastroesophageal reflux (GER). Most of the cases will respond to esophageal dilatation. However, some are refractory to dilatation and require surgical resection. The impact of CES on the response to and efficacy of dilatation is not known. The cause of refractory strictures is said to be related to GER, age at diagnosis, and delayed initiation of dilatation [22, 24, 25]. A *retrospective study* by the first author was conducted between January 2006 to December 2014 at the pediatric surgery department of armed forces hospitals southern region in Saudi Arabia after being approved by the local research and Ethics committee [3] In contrast to the CES group in that study all cases of the non-CES group showed significantly a better response and effect to dilatations. It was concluded that CES should be added as a possible important cause of refractory stricture (whether anastomotic or distal) after EA repair and it may partially explain why some of these strictures are refractory to dilatations (refer to Table 6.1). In this table, the statistical analysis of data was done by using SPSS 22 for IBM program. The data was described as mean [min/max] for quantitative data and numbers and percentage for qualitative data. Independent sample t-test was used to compare two groups in quantitative data and Chi-square test was used for qualitative data. P is considered significant if $\leq$0.05. Table 6.1 shows that the data analyzed including age at first presentation, number of dilatation sessions, excellent response to dilatation, refectory response, very effective response

Table 6.1 Comparison between results of balloon dilatations for EA/TEF with symptomatic AS and CES associated with EA

Item	EA/TEF with symptomatic AS N = 58/126 (46%)	CES associated with EA N = 16/126 (12.7%)	P value
Post operative symptomatic stenosis	58/126	13/126 (3 cases excluded)[a]	<0.001
Sex	Male: 32 Female: 26	5 8	0.43
Age at first presentation	Mean: 37.6 months Range: 1 month to 10 years	49.3 days 1–60 days	<0.001
Number of sessions	106 for 58 patients	106 for 13 patients	<0.001
Sessions interval	2 weeks	2 weeks	
Excellent response	37 (63.8%)	2 (15.4%)	<0.002
Satisfactory response	20 (34.5%)	4 (30.8%)	0.91
Fair response	0 (0.0 %)	0 (0.0%)	0.00
Refractory response	1 (1.7%)	7 (50%)	<0.001
Very effective	57 (98.2%)	4 (30.8%)	<0.001
Effective	1 (1.7%)	2 (15.4%)	0.17
Ineffective	– (0.0%)	7 (50%)	<0.001
Perforation	0.00%	0.00%	0.00

EA Esophageal atresia, *TEF* tracheoesophageal fistula
Excellent response (one session), Satisfactory (up to 5 sessions), Fair (ʾ5 sessions)
Very effective = No dysphagia, Effective = dysphagia to special types of food
[a]3 patients excluded, 2 patients with gastric pull-up due to TBR with cartilage in the whole lower pouches, 1 patient having TBR without cartilage with asymptomatic stenosis

and ineffective response are all highly significant. This confirms the fact that CES associated with EA is an important risk factor inducing a refractory stricture.

Tovar and Fragoso [26] performed a study in 2013 which illustrated that GER is common in EA/TEF and does not seem to improve with medical treatment. The esophagus is persistently defective having abnormal extrinsic and intrinsic innervations. Moreover, the motor function and sphincters are defective. Around 50% of the patients suffer chronic GER that ends up with a Barrette esophagitis. Fundoplication becomes necessary in 40% of cases especially in cases with long gap EA and in refractory anastomotic stenosis. Esophageal carcinoma is a potential risk with a 50-fold more frequent in EA than in the regular population. Fundoplication in those cases is fairly difficult to perform and tends to fail in almost one-fifth of those children. This needs close observation and reoperation whenever necessary. Redo surgery may be required in 18.1% of the cases [26].

Indications of Anti-reflux Surgery

The main indication for fundoplication is failure of a well-conducted medical treatment based on posture, diet, and appropriate antacids as well as prokinetics. This course of conservative management should not be prolonged for more than

2–3 weeks. Persistent vomiting, failure to thrive (FTT), life threatening respiratory disease, acute life threatening events (ALTE), repeated aspiration, recurrent pneumonia, or severe esophagitis require antireflux surgery. Some patients do not have expectations for improvement with conservative management and require fundoplication primarily. Cases of refractory anastomotic stenosis require fundoplication for better results of dilatations [26]. This also applies for cases of CES if initial dilatation is not successful [3, 12]. There is a direct relation between GER and refractory stenosis and surgical indications are clear in such cases. Cases of pure atresia and long-gap EA have their anastomosis under severe tension leading to GER. Foker's technique for esophageal lengthening is followed by GER and require fundoplication in 100% of cases. Cases of EA associated with duodenal atresia have a bad sphincter, poor esophageal peristalsis, poor gastric emptying, pyloric insufficiency and biliary reflux requiring fundoplication [26].

Gastrostomy

Gastrostomy tube (GT) is a tube passed into the stomach through the abdominal wall for enteral feeding. It is frequently used in cases of CES with severe stricture or major esophageal dysmotility. The first successful gastrostomy in humans was done in 1876 by Verneoil as cited by Abu-Hilal et al. [27]. Stamm in 1894, described one of the most common techniques commonly practiced nowadays [28]. The percutaneous endoscopic gastrostomy (PEG) was introduced by Gauderer et al. in 1980 [29].

Indications for Gastrostomy Tube (GT) Insertion

These include difficulty in swallowing as in cerebral palsy, severe facial trauma, luminal obstruction by benign or malignant strictures and hyper catabolic states [30]. Beside nutritional support the GT can be used for giving medications and for gastric decompression. If a nasogastric tube (NGT) is required for feeding for more than a period of 4–6 weeks, then a GT is indicated [31]. Trans-gastric, intermittent feeding is preferred. In our studies on 12 patients with CES associated with EA/TEF [3, 12], gastrostomies were performed due to severe stricture and the development of the ominous triad of GER, dysmotility and severe stricture in 9 patients. Gastrostomies are more likely to be required in cases of CES associated with EA rather than the isolated type.

Types of Gastrostomies There are three types of gastrostomies; the percutaneous fluoroscopic gastrostomy, percutaneous endoscopic gastrostomy (PEG), and surgical Stamm gastrostomy. Although PEG is already known to be safer than the surgical one yet it has some limitations. It might be impossible to pass the endoscope due to benign or malignant strictures [32]. The most common cases requiring gastrostomies in our experience are those with difficulty in swallowing in cases of cerebral palsy with or without GER and cases of severe esophageal stricture after operation of EA with or without CES. Most of these cases required a surgical procedure since the accessibility to the stomach through the esophagus was not possible. Also; many of those cases will require a concomitant fundoplication. So, our preferred approach is an open surgical classical Stamm gastrostomy if a fundoplication is required. If a fundoplication is not required, a laparoscopic assisted gastrostomy is performed. We usually use a Foley's catheter size 12–16 Fr (according to age) till a gastrostomy track is well formed within 6 weeks to 2 month period then replaced by a ballooned button gastrostomy. So, surgical gastrostomy is our option when there is need for laparotomy and when there is severe stricture making the stomach not accessible through the esophagus. When laparotomy is not required and a gastrostomy is required alone due to prolonged requirement of NGT feeding, then a laparoscopic assisted Stamm gastrostomy can be performed [33].

The endoscopic gastrostomy is usually performed by endoscopist physicians and requires specific materials and tubes. The unavailability of such materials for pediatric patients may be a factor to use the surgical gastrostomy more frequently in some cases in children. PEG is also not devoid of complications [34].

Some recommendations proposed by Ansilmo et al. in 2013 to avoid complications of the gastrostomy are: a punctiform opening in the anterior gastric wall between the greater and lesser curvatures, use of a double purse–string non-absorbable suture, fixation of the gastric wall to the abdominal wall using non-absorbable sutures without tension, proper fixation of the tube to the anterior abdominal wall to prevent displacement, Post operative fasting period of at least 24 h, testing the patency of the gastrostomy tube with saline solution and check for any intraperitoneal spillage, and testing the tube with dextrose 5% drip the second post-operative day. Ensure compliance of the patient for enteral feeding [35]. We usually start milk feeding on the 3rd day postoperatively with instructions to push little water to wash the milk off the tube.

We had an experience with 135 surgical Stamm gastrostomies in neurologically impaired (NI) patients. A total of 112 patients were referred for gastrostomy due to oral feeding difficulties (FD). Our protocol is to go for a complete barium swallow and meal. If there is GER, we will proceed for a fundoplication together with a Stamm gastrostomy. Initially we used a complete wrap (Nissen Fundoplication), but later we shifted to the partial anterior wrap (Thal fundoplication). The latter is easier, with comparative results and less complications in our hands than Nissen fundoplication in NI patients with esophageal dysmotility. Our results and complications of the Stamm gastrostomy with fundoplication in NI patients are shown in Table 6.2.

Gastrostomy Complications

Early in the course, two patients had concomitant pyloroplasty with fundoplication due to delayed gastric emptying discovered by preoperative barium study. One of the patients had perforation of the pyloroplasty by the GT. We stopped doing pyloroplasties since then and we found that these patients with delayed gastric emptying improve alone after fundoplication. Mortality whether early or late in cases of NI patients are not related to gastrostomy surgery itself but to the bad general conditions of the patients. The most common minor complication of gastrostomy was the granuloma formation and mucosal prolapse (Fig. 6.1). Most of these patients respond to local application of silver nitrate. The problem of external leakage, skin infection and excoriation was managed in the emergency department by keeping

Table 6.2 NI patients having GER and oral feeding difficulties (94/136 = 69%) requiring fundoplication and GT in 15 year-period

Sex	Male: 49	
	Female: 45	
Age	Infants (up to 12 mos) N = 50	
	Range: 1.5–12 mos, Mean: 6.4 mos	
	Children (above one year) N = 44	
	Range: 1.5–12 years, Mean: 5 years	
Operations	# Nissen/tamm gastrostomy	27
	# Nissen/Stamm gastrostomy/cricomyotomy	1
	# Nissen/Stamm gastrostomy/pyloroplasty	2
	# Gastrostomy followed by Nissen	6
	# Thal/Stamm gastrostomy	58
Complications	# Early mortality within 1 month	1
	# Early perforation of the pyloroplasty by the GT	1
	# Later mortality	3
	# Adhesion intestinal obstruction	2
	# gastrostomy fistula closed surgically	2
	# granuloma	9
	# Leakage outside	5
	# Leakage intraperitoneal	2
	# Dislodgment	4
	# Gastrostomy revision	3

NI neurologically impaired, *Mos* months, *GT* gastrostomy tube
NB: mortality was related to the primary disease and not to the surgical procedure

Fig. 6.1 Gastrostomy site with excoriation due to partial mucosal prolapse and leakage

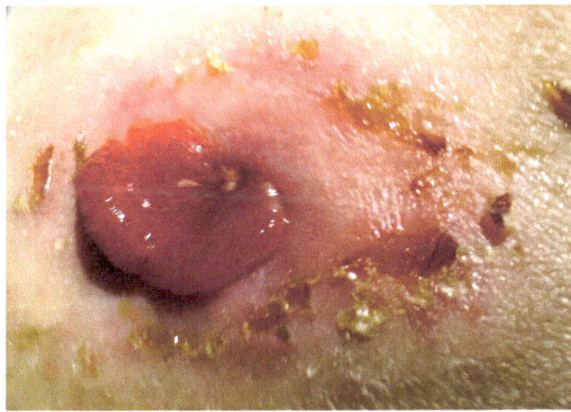

Table 6.3 NI patients having oral feeding difficulties without GER (42/136 = 31%) requiring GT only in 15 year-period

Sex	Male: 30	
	Female: 12	
Age	Infants (more than 1–12 mos): N = 16	
	Range = 2–12 mos, Mean = 7.8 mos	
	Children (up to 12 years): N = 26	
	Range = 1.5–11 years, Mean = 6.8 years	
Operations	Stamm gastrostomy	18
	Post fundoplication gastrostomy	2
	Gastrostomy followed by fundoplication	6
	Laparoscopic assisted gastrostomy	16
Complications	# gastrostomy fistula requiring surgery	1
	# GER	6
	# Gastrostomy revision	1
	# Granuloma	4
	# Excoriation	3
	# Dislodgment	2

NI neurologically impaired, *Mos* months, *GT* gastrostomy tube

the patient fasting, giving intravenous fluids and removing the GT for a period of 6–8 h to allow the gastrostomy opening to get smaller. Then the same size GT or button is repositioned when the gastrostomy opening is tight over the tube. Other gastrostomy complications include pressure ulcers, tube occlusion (frequent), colon perforation, buried bumper syndrome (BBS in cases of PEG), Dislodgement and persistent gastrostomy fistula requiring surgery after removal of the gastrostomy.

Our results of other NI patients without GER who had Stamm gastrostomy only are shown in Table 6.3. In this group, we used to do open Stamm gastrostomy without fundoplication. However, two patients required gastrostomy after a fundoplication. Also, 6 patients required fundoplication after gastrostomy due to massive GER. Subsequently, all patients requiring gastrostomy alone were done laparoscopically assisted. The main problem then in these patients was the development of GER requiring reoperation for fundoplication. Whether to proceed for fundoplication with gastrostomy even in cases without GER or not is a controversial issue. Nonfatal and minor complications of gastrostomy are almost the same in all cases with neurological impairment.

Role of Gastrostomy in CES

A gastrostomy is more likely to be required for cases of pure EA waiting for delayed primary repair. It is required in cases of CES associated with EA and/or TEF rather than cases of isolated CES. This is true when there is severe stricture, major esophageal dysmotility with difficulty of oral feeding and significant GER not responding to medical treatment. The typical scenario is a failure of dilatation of the stricture, failure of antireflux measures together with esophageal motility problem. Patients with this ominous triad (stricture, GER and dysmotility) will actually require a partial fundoplication together with a Stamm gastrostomy to improve the general condition of the patient and treat GER which may be the cause of the bad general condition, bad chest, secondary esophageal dysmotility and refractory strictures. After surgery, retrial of dilatation is then practiced. If this fails then resection of the stricture is advised. Most of the cases will need post-resection esophageal dilatations again (Table 6.4). The gastrostomy together with a partial anterior fundoplication is essential in these difficult cases of CES. This allows regular gastrostomy feeding, chest improvement, prevention of GER and the possibility of a successful dilatation after GER control. Moreover, gastrostomy will allow retrograde stricture dilatation in difficult cases. The gastrostomy was done as a temporary procedure and finally removed with improvement of the general condition of the patient and successful oral feeding with disappearance of dysphagia.

The dilatation courses might be protracted but this might save the patient own esophagus instead of esophageal replacement with all of its complications. There is always a concern about the danger of long term usage of fluoroscopy or flexible endoscopy both of which require general anesthesia in children. However, this should be balanced against the complications of replacing the patient own esophagus. It is always said that the patient's own esophagus is the best conduit for food. We had 4 patients with protracted courses of dilatations. Eventually they are doing well with a normal life style and eating everything without dysphagia [3, 12].

The Antireflux Surgery in Pediatrics

More than 60% of patients with GER will resolve spontaneously within one years of age [36]. Gastroesophageal reflux disease (GERD) develops when symptoms fail to disappear, or complications develop. Complications include failure to thrive (FTT), respiratory problems, stridor, esophagitis and esophageal strictures.

Although spontaneous resolution of GER occurs in most infants, certain debilitating nutritional effects in the early months of life may have a life time consequences especially in the developing brain [37].

FTT is a major problem in neonates and infants because this is the time when the brain needs to grow and waiting for a period of 1–2 years for the LES to develop is unwise. If other causes of FTT are excluded, then full antireflux measures should be started.

Barium swallow and meal, milk scan, and upper gastrointestinal esophagoscopy are important aid for diagnosis of GERD. The 24-h reflux index is approved as the most specific and sensitive predictor for pathologic reflux especially when a dual probe is used [38–40]. However, it is unable to detect non-acidic reflux which can contribute to acute and chronic respiratory problems [41]. Recently, multi-channel intraluminal impedance will assess the velocity and direction of liquid and gas flow through the esophagus [38].

Table 6.4 Cases of CES associated with EA/and or TEF requiring fundoplication and gastrostomy (11/16) (68.8%)

No	Sex	Type of CES and site	Risk factors for GT	Treatment	Age	Outcome
1	F	FMD Distal, sparing, GEJ	Severe AS, GER +++ and major dysmotility Difficult feeding	ARM, dilatations myotomy/Nissen/GT/ dilatations Resection, anastomosis	3 mos 6 mos 9 mos	Improved
2	F	TBR Cartilage + anastomotic	Pure EA FTT/GER/aspiration Later major dysmotility	Gastrostomy Delayed primary repair ARM/Thal/GT gastric pull-up	3 days 6 mos 10 mos	Improved
3	F	TBR No cartilage Anastomotic	Stricture, GER +++/dysmotility/FTT	ARM/dilatations Thal/GT Resection primary anastomosis dilatations	3 mos 6 mos 9 mos	Improved
4	F	FMD anastomotic	Stricture/GER +++/dysmotility/FTT	ARM/dilatations Thal/GT Diverticulectomy dilatations	3 mos 6 mos 14 mos	Improved
5	M	TBR Whole LP	Pure EA Major dysmotility/GER++	GT Delayed primary repair Cut Collis Nissen fundoplication Gastric pull up	3 days 9 mos 11 mos 12 mos	Mortality due to severe sepsis
6	M	TBR Cartilage + anastomotic	Moderate AS Major dysmotility	Single dilatation Thal/GT/lower myectomy	1 mos 6 weeks	Improved

7	F	TBR Cartilage + anastomotic	Stricture, GER+++ Major dysmotility	ARM/dilatations Thal/GT/Dilatations Resection primary anastomosis Dilatations × 20 sessions	2 mos 4 mos 7 mos To 60 mos	Improved
8	F	TBR Cartilage + anastomotic	Stricture, GER, dysmotility	Dilatation/ARM Thal/GT/Dilatation Resection/anastomosis Dilatation × 22 sessions	2 mos 4 mos 7 mos Up to 96	Improved
9	M	TBR Cartilage + anastomotic	Major dysmotility	Thal/GT + Lower myectomy	1.5 mos	Improved
10	M	? TBR Distal	GER/dysmotility/stricture/recurrent TEF	ARM/Thal + GT Refractory distal stricture esophagostomy	1 mos 24 mos	Mortality
11	F	FMD (distal)	GER/dysmotility/distal stricture/ Fanconi's anemia	Dilatation, myectomy/Thal and GT	1 mos	Mortality at 3 years

ARM antireflux measures, *GT* gastrostomy tube, *GER* gastroesophageal reflux, *mos* months

The main lines of medical treatment include head up position, dietary thickeners, small frequent feeds, antacids like H2-blockers and proton pump inhibitors (PPI), surface barrier agents and prokinetics. The North American Society for Pediatric Gastroenterology, Hepatology and Nutrition (NASPGHAN) and the European Society for Pediatric Gastroenterology, Hepatology and Nutrition (ESPGHAN) have concluded that there is insufficient evidence to justify the routine use of prokinetics. Esomeprazole (Nexium) has been approved in USA for short term treatment of GERD with esophagitis [41, 42]. Esomeprazole will not prevent respiratory problems and recurrent apneic episodes in infants and neonates. The decrease of acid exposure will increase non-acidic reflux resulting in persistence of vomiting and recurrent respiratory symptoms [43]. Thickening of formula feeds may reduce frank emesis but does not reduce GER. There is no quality data to support that more frequent but smaller volume feeding reduce GER. A 60° head up position increases GER compared to prone position. However, the prone position is dangerous as it may lead to sudden infant death syndrome. Also, no significant difference has been found between the flat and head-elevation prone position [9]. Only anti-reflux surgery can prevent recurrent aspiration pneumonia, recurrent apneic attacks and chronic respiratory problems [41, 45].

Anti-reflux surgery is indicated after failure of medical management like in cases of FTT, most respiratory symptoms and esophagitis. However, fundoplication without a trial of medical therapy may be performed in selected cases including cases of GERD requiring gastrostomy, those with ALTEs, Barrett's esophagitis, and esophageal stricture. Finally, cases of congenital hiatal defects and post Esophageal atresia (EA) repair may require fundoplication as the initial therapy [41, 44].

Results of surgery are better in cases of primary GERD than in high risk candidates like neurologic impairment, congenital diaphragmatic hernia, and chronic respiratory conditions or repaired EA [38, 44]. The outcome is variable in the literature. Excellent results have been reported with improvement of symptoms and weight gain [41]. Other reports showed poor results after fundoplication in young infants with high failure rate [46, 47]. Laparoscopic Nissen fundoplication can be performed safely and effectively in small children weighing less than 5 kg with similar outcomes and rates of complications as those reported in older children [48]. It is also reported that in the long term, open and laparoscopic Thal fundoplication have similarly good outcomes [49].

In conclusion, surgery for GERD in infants less than 12 months of age is a controversial issue. Only infants with failed medical treatment and those with life-threatening complications of GERD, recurrent pneumonia, growth failure and ongoing ventilator-dependence secondary to recurrent aspiration are candidates for fundoplication. Although Nissen fundoplication is now well established as a treatment option in selected cases of GERD in children, its role in neonates and infants is unclear and only few reports have been published [39, 41, 42, 44, 45] Thal fundoplication in neonates and infants is even less reported in the literature and its role needs to be further investigated in this group of patients.

The fundoplication is highly effective and provides a definitive treatment for GERD [50]. It is mentioned that a floppy Nissen fundoplication is the most preferred option for cases requiring fundoplication. The fundus of the stomach is wrapped around the distal esophagus for 360°. It has become the operation for the surgical treatment of GERD both in children and in adults (IPEG guide lines 2009). The original Nissen was wrapping the distal esophagus for a distance of 4–5 cm. This length was then reduced to 1–2 cm to avoid a tight Nissen and dysphagia [51].

However, there are some difficulties regarding Nissen fundoplication. Esophageal dysmotility, small gastric fundus, an obtuse angle of Hiss, a short esophagus and possible migration of the wrap into the chest are factors against this option. In this situation the partial anterior wrap (Thal or Boix-Ochoa) [52] or posterior (Toupet) [53] are preferred. This involves 270° wrapping of the gastric fundus around the lower esophagus. The partial wrap is designed to prevent dysphagia in cases with esophageal motility disorders. It is claimed that the partial wraps has worse long term results. Esposito et al. showed that there is no statistical significance in the outcome between laparoscopic Nissen, Toupet and Thal fundoplications in neurologically normal children [54]. Kubiak et al. in a prospective randomized study compared between Nissen fundoplication and Thal in children. The Nissen fundoplication had a significantly lower recurrence rate than the Thal (5.9% versus 15.5%) in neurologically impaired patients. However, there was no such significant difference in normal children. The incidence of post-operative dysphagia was similar in both groups, but significantly more patients in the Nissen group required reoperation for severe dysphagia (11.8% versus 2.4%) [55].

The requirement of a pyloroplasty together with the fundoplication is a controversial issue. The question is whether to do a concomitant pyloroplasty with the fundoplication or not. Maxson et al. showed that there is no deference in terms of recurrence of symptoms or requirements of reoperation. Moreover, postoperative complications have been reported to be higher when pyloroplasty was added to the fundoplication [56]. Now it is a common practice that pyloroplasty is not performed with fundoplication [57].

The addition of a fundoplication to a gastrostomy tube requested in a neurologically impaired child for feeing is a controversial issue. A barium contrast study is usually performed preoperatively. If GER is diagnosed, many of the surgeons prefer to go for a fundoplication with the gastrostomy. Others will not do that due to a poorer prognosis of a fundoplication in these groups of patients [58]. However, reflux-related hospital admissions for neurologically impaired children who underwent Nissen fundoplication were reduced compared to hospital admissions before fundoplication [45].

Complications of the Anti-reflux Surgery

Intraoperative complications include bleeding, perforation of the esophagus, stomach, or intestine, vagus nerve injury and pneumothorax [59, 60]. Initial postoperative complications include dysphagia and gas bloat. Gas bloat is relieved by a NGT insertion or opening the gastrostomy tube if present. Dysphagia usually resolves within 3 weeks after surgery. However, Nissen fundoplication has a higher rate of severe dysphagia that requires reoperation in comparison to Thal or Toupet [55]. Long term complications include failed fundoplication with recurrent symptoms, dysphagia and abnormal pH studies. This is more common in NI than in neurologically normal patients (12% versus 2%) [61]. The most common causes of failed fundoplication are disruption of the wrap, wrap slippage, a sliding hernia with intact wrap, too tight or too long wrap, intrathoracic herniation of the wrap and twisted wrap [62]. A redo surgery is feasible but challenging due to severe adhesions and the need to mobilize the esophagus, crural repair, and wrap reformation [60, 63].

We had experience with 199 cases of open fundoplications over a 15-year period (until May 2014). Recently we are performing fundoplication laparoscopically which will not be discussed here. Open fundoplication has been done for both NI (94 patients) and non NI patients (105 patients), the indications of which are shown in Tables 6.5 and 6.6 respectively. A total of 136 of NI patients have been referred mainly for gastrostomy insertion and/or an anti-reflux surgery. The main indication for a gastrostomy tube was difficulty in feeding. A total of 94 patients were offered a fundoplication together with a GT due to associated GER. The remaining 42 patients were offered A GT only since there was no GER upon contrast study.

Table 6.5 Fundoplication in NI patients (94/199 = 47.2%)

Patient	Indication for surgery	Type of surgery	Total number
NI	Difficulty in feeding, GERD, FTT	Nissen fundoplication + Stamm gastrostomy	21
NI	Difficulty in feeding, GERD, FTT	Thal fundoplication + Stamm gastrostomy	55
NI	Difficulty in feeding, no GERD, FTT	Stamm gastrostomy followed by Nissen fundoplication due to massive GER not responding to conservative treatment	4
NI	Difficulty in feeding, No GERD, FTT	Stamm gastrostomy followed by Thal fundoplication due to massive GER not responding to conservative treatment	2
NI	Massive GERD, recurrent vomiting and chest infection Failed medical treatment	Nissen fundoplication followed by gastrostomy due to FTT	2
NI	Massive GERD, recurrent vomiting and chest infection Failed medical treatment	Thal fundoplication followed by gastrostomy due to FTT	1
NI	Massive GERD, recurrent vomiting and chest infection Failed medical treatment	Nissen fundoplication	9

NI neurologically impaired, *FTT* failure to thrive, *GERD* gastroesophageal reflux disease

Table 6.6 Fundoplication in non NI patients (105/199 = 52.8%)

Category	Indications for fundoplication	Type of surgery	Number
Primary GER	Failed medical treatment FTT ALTE Intolerance to feeds Thoracic stomach HH	Nissen Thal	17 24
Post EA repair	GER, dysmotility, stricture Intolerance to feed FTT Severe pulmonary disease	Nissen ± GT Thal ± GT	11 17
CES (with EA/ TEF) CES (isolated)	GER, dysmotility, stricture Failed medical treatment Failed dilatation Intolerance to feed Achalasia-like/dysphagia failed dilatation/ TBR	Nissen + GT Thal + GT Primary resection Anastomosis/ Nissen	1 10 5
Cardiac achalasia	Dysphagia Respiratory problems Failed dilatation	Nissen/myotomy Thal/myectomy	6 4
Corrosive ingestion	GER/severe stricture	Nissen/GT	10

NI neurologically impaired, *FTT* failure to thrive, *ALTE* acute life threatening events, *HH* Hiatus hernia, *GER* Gastroesophageal reflux, *GT* gastrostomy tube, *TBR* Tracheobronchial remnants

A consultation for the ENT surgical team was usually required preoperatively to assess the upper airway. Ten patients out of 94 NI patients had stridor due to reflux laryngitis; two of them had already tracheostomy for that. Stridor improved gradually after fundoplication and the tracheostomy could be removed safely in the remaining two. Only 12/94 (12.8%) NI patients were referred due to severe GER which did not respond to medical management. All of them had a fundoplication procedure. However three of those required a gastrostomy subsequently due to failure to thrive despite of improvement of GER symptoms and signs. The remaining 42 NI patients had GT only. Initially we used to do a classical Stamm gastrostomy. The last 16 patients were done laparoscopically assisted. Six patients subsequently developed massive GER and required a fundoplication procedure. The main symptoms in our group of patients were FTT, intolerance to feed requiring GT for feeding and respiratory problems. Ten patients had stridor due to reflux laryngitis. Few had symptoms of reflux esophagitis. The most common diagnostic tools for GERD in our institution were esophagogram, upper gastrointestinal series, gastric emptying studies, esophagogastroduodenoscopy, esophageal biopsy and histology.

Only four patients had peptic stricture. One of them (a hemophilia patient) had significant bleeding not responding to full antireflux measures for months. Barium and flexible endoscopic studies confirmed the diagnosis of reflux esophagitis and hiatus hernia. There were 17 patients who had concomitant hiatus hernia (a moderate sized hernia) and 3 patients born with thoracic stomach (A major hiatal hernia or a congenital short esophagus). Eight NI patients out of seventeen had hiatus hernia while in non NI patients, 9 had hiatus hernia and three had thoracic stomach. For cases of EA/TEF we had a total of 17 cases that required a fundoplication after failure of aggressive anti reflux measures.

Fundoplication and CES Associated with EA

Eleven patients of EA associated with CES required fundoplication and GT (Table 6.4). The main indication of gastrostomy was inability to feed due to the ominous triad of stricture, dysmotility and GER. This is the worthiest situation a surgeon may face in the management of EA associated with CES. The option was to replace the esophagus in most of the cases. However the decision was to go through the steps of aggressive antireflux measures, balloon dilatations, fundoplication with gastrostomy, redilatation, resection if refractory and finally prolonged courses of balloon dilatation with an interval of 1–2 weeks between dilatation sessions. With this protocol we could avoid esophageal replacement. Patients are enjoying a normal life and eating everything without dysphagia. We had two mortalities out of the 11 patients. The first mortality was a case of pure atresia and TBR with cartilage involving the whole lower esophagus. The patient had gastrostomy, delayed primary repair and later a gastric pullup due to major esophageal dysmotility and massive GER. Histopathological examination of the resected lower esophageal pouch showed TBR with cartilage. This patient died of severe sepsis at the age of one year. The second mortality was a male triplet with EA/TEF who had a primary repair on the 3rd day of life. On the 7th post-operative day he had contrast study which showed GER and doubtful area of distal CES sparing the GEJ. Feeding was started with full anti reflux measures. He had a massive aspiration on the 15th postoperative day which ended up with a major brain damage. A repeat of esophagogram confirmed the diagnosis of distal CES sparing the GEJ and recurrent TEF (Fig. 4.3a–c). He was offered a Thal fundoplication and a GT. The stricture was undilatable in two occasions with failure to pass the guide wire even endoscopically. The case was discussed with the parents and it was agreed to go for an esophagostomy rather than a major surgery due to severe brain damage. We learned from this case that:

1. CES can be easily missed in the initial esophagogram in the neonatal period
2. It can progress so rapidly to a very tight stricture within days
3. It can be too severe to endanger the life of the patient in the neonatal period
4. GER and esophageal dysmotility are co factors to endanger life.
5. It is possible that CES can be a cause of recurrent TEF due to distal obstruction which is another co factor endangering life.
6. If the diagnosis is missed and mortality or a major disability happens in the neonatal period or early in infancy then the real incidence of CES is never known.
7. Early diagnosis of CES in the neonatal period and proper management can be lifesaving.

A high index of suspicion should be practiced during the initial esophagogram after EA repair. If CES is suspected, feeding can be started with full anti reflux measures including pump drip feeding or trans-pyloric NGT feeding. Keeping the patient NPO together with TPN for 3–4 weeks post EA repair till it is possible to go for balloon dilatation is another option. Balloon dilatation 3–4 weeks after EA repair is safe and is both diagnostic and therapeutic.

We are using open Thal fundoplication for more than 12 years with good results.

Laparoscopic Nissen is now widely used [64]. Esposito et al. showed that laparoscopic fundoplication was feasible even in pediatric patients less than one year of age [65].

A Collis plasty may be required for lengthening of the intrabdominal esophagus followed by fundoplication [66]. The wrap fails in a range from 10 to 50% with an average of 18.1% in cases of EA versus 7% in regular refluxers [26].

Long segment CES has been reported, the earliest of which is that reported by Bluestone et al. in 1969 [67]. In that case the stenosis continued to taper till the GEJ. Multiple CES have been also reported [68, 69]. In such rare and difficult cases, the standard procedures such as resection and anastomosis, enucleation and myectomy are not possible. In such severe varieties, cardioplasty Collis gastroplasty-Nissen fundoplication, stricturotomy [69] and esophageal replacement [67] have been described. In such cases the surgeon should have an open mind and use whatever is available to him while maintaining basic surgical principles. The surgical procedures have to be tailored based on the individual cases for an optimum result [69].

References

1. Al Shamrani J, Quesnel S, Pierrot S, Couloigner V. Endoscopic balloon dilatation of esophageal strictures in children. Int J Pediatr Otorhinolaryngol. 2011;75(11):1376–9. https://doi.org/10.1016/j.ijporl.2011.07.031.
2. Poddar U, Thaba BR. Benign esophageal stricture in infants and children: results of Savary-Gilliard bougie dilatation in 107 Indian children. Gastrointest Endosc. 2001;54(4):480–4. https://doi.org/10.1067/mge.2001.118253.
3. Ibrahim AHM, Bazeed MF, Jamil S, Hamad HA, Abdel Raheem IM, Ashraf I. Management of congenital esophageal stenosis associated with esophageal atresia and its impact on postoperative esophageal stricture. Ann Pediatr Surg. 2016;12:36–4. https://doi.org/10.1097/01.XPS.0000482656 06000.84.
4. Romeo E, Foschia F, de Angelis P, Caldaro T, di Abriola GF, Gambitta R, et al. Endoscopic management of congenital esophageal stenosis. J Pediatr Surg. 2011;46:838–41. https://doi.org/10.1016/j.jpedsurg.2011.02.010.
5. Usui N, Kamata S, Kawahara H, Sawai T, Nakajima K, Soh H, Okada A. Usefulness of endoscopic ultrasonography in the diagnosis of congenital esophageal stenosis. J Pediatr Surg. 2002;37:1744–6. https://doi.org/10.1053/jpsu.2002.36711.
6. Kouchi K, Yoshida H, Matsunage T, Ohtsuka Y, Nagatake E, Satoh Y, Terue K, Mitsunage T, et al. Endosonographic evaluation in two children with esophageal stenosis. J Pediatr Surg. 2002;37:934–6. https://doi.org/10.1053/jpsu.2002.32921.

7. Teuri K, Saito T, Mitsunaga T, Nakata M, Yoshida H. Endoscopic management for congenital esophageal stenosis: a systematic review. World J Gastrointest Endosc. 2015;7(3):183–91. https://doi.org/10.4253/wjge.v7.i3.183.
8. Baird R, Laberge JM, Lévesque D. Anastomotic stricture after esophageal atresia repair: a critical review of recent literature. Eur J Pediatr Surg. 2013;23:204–13. https://doi.org/10.105 5/s-0033-1347917.
9. Shorter NA, Mooney DP, Vaccaro TJ, Sargent SK. Hydrostatic balloon dilatation of congenital esophageal stenosis associated with esophageal atresia. J Pediatr Surg. 2000;35:1742–5. https://doi.org/10.1053/jpsu.2000.19238.
10. Kawahara H, Imura K, Yagi M, Kubota A. Clinical characteristic of congenital oesophageal stenosis distal to associated oesophageal atresia. Surgery. 2001;129:29–3.
11. Yeung CK, Spitz L, Brereton RJ, Kiely EM, Leak J. Congenital esophageal stenosis due to tracheobronchial remnants: a rare but important association with esophageal atresia. J Pediatr Surg. 1992;27:852–5.
12. Ibrahim AH, Al Malki TA, Hamza AF, Bahnasy AF. Congenital esophageal stenosis associated with esophageal atresia: new concepts. Pediatr Surg Int. 2007;23:533–7. https://doi.org/10.1007/s00383-007-1927-5.
13. Amae S, Nio M, Kamiyama T, Ishii T, Yoshida S, Hayashi Y, et al. Clinical characteristics and management of congenital esophageal stenosis: a report on 14 cases. J Pediatr Surg. 2003;38:565–70. https://doi.org/10.1053/jpsu.2003.50123.
14. Neuman B, Bender TM. Esophageal atresia/tracheoesophageal fistula and associated congenital stenosis. Pediatr Radiol. 1997;27:530–4. https://doi.org/10.1007/s002470050174.
15. Fékété CN, Backer AD, Jacob SL. Congenital esophageal stenosis, a review of 20 cases. Pediatr Surg Int. 1987;2:86–92. https://doi.org/10.1007/BF00174179.
16. Neilson IR, Croitoru DP, Guttman FM, Yossef S, Laberge JM. Distal congenital esophageal stenosis associated with esophageal atresia. J Pediatr Surg. 1991;26:478–82. https://doi.org/10.1016/0022-3468(91)90999-A.
17. Maeda K, Hisamatsu C, Hasegawa T, Tanaka H, Okita Y. Circular myectomy for the treatment of congenital esophageal stenosis owing to tracheobronchial remnants. J Pediatr Surg. 2004;39:1765–8. https://doi.org/10.1016/j.jpedsurg.2004.08.016.
18. Saito T, Ise K, Kawahara Y, Yamashita M, Shimizu H, Suzuki H, Gotoh M. Congenital esophageal stenosis because of tracheobronchial remnants and treated by circular myectomy. J Pediatr Surg. 2008;43:583–5. https://doi.org/10.1016/j.jpedsurg.2007.11.017.
19. Martinez-Ferro M, Rubio M, Piaggio L, Laje P. Thoracoscopic approach for congenital esophageal stenosis. J Pediatr Surg. 2006;41:E5–7. https://doi.org/10.1016/j.jpedsurg.2006.06.022.
20. Deshpande AV, Shun A. Laparoscopic treatment of congenital esophageal stenosis due to tracheobronchial remnants in a child. J Laparoendosc Adv Surg. 2009;19:107–9. https://doi.org/10.1089/lap.2008.0070.
21. Suzuhigashi M, Kaji T, Nogushi H, Muto M, Goto M, Mukai M, Nakame M, et al. Current characteristics and management of congenital esophageal stenosis: 40 consecutive cases from a multicenter study in the Kyushu area of Japan. Pediatr Surg Int. 2017;33:1035–40. https://doi.org/10.1007/s00383-017-4133-0.
22. Antoniou D, Soutis M, Christopoulos-Geroulanos G. Anastomotic strictures following esophageal atresia repair: a 20-year experience with endoscopic balloon dilatation. J Pediatr Gastroenterol Nutr. 2010;51:464–7. https://doi.org/10.1097/MPG.0b013e3181d682ac.
23. Said M, Mekki M, Golli F, Hafsa C, Braham R, Braham R, et al. Balloon dilatation of anastomotic strictures secondary to surgical repair of esophageal atresia. Br J Radiol. 2003;76:26–31. https://doi.org/10.1259/bjr/64412147.
24. Kim IO, Yeon KM, Kim WS, Park KW, Kim JH, Han MC. Perforation complicating balloon dilatation of esophageal strictures in infants and children. Radiology. 1993;189:741–4. https://doi.org/10.1148/radiology.189.3.8234699.
25. Chittmittrapap S, Spitz L, Kiely EM, Brereton RJ. Anastomotic stricture following repair of esophageal atresia. J Pediatr Surg. 1990;25:508–11. https://doi.org/10.1016/0022-3468(90)90561-M.

26. Tovar JA, Fragoso AC. Gastroesophageal reflux after repair of esophageal atresia. Eur J Pediatr Surg. 2013;23:175–81. https://doi.org/10.1055/s-0033-1347911.
27. Abu-Hilal M, Hemandas AK, McPhail M, Jain G, Panagiotopoulou I, Scibelli T, Johnson CDA. Comparative analysis of safety and efficacy of different methods of tube placement for enteral feeding following major pancreatic resection. a non-randomized study. J Pancreas. 2010;11(1):8–13.
28. Stamm M. Gastrostomy: a new method. Med Newsl. 1894;65:324.
29. Gauderer MW, Ponsky J, Izant RJ. Gastrostomy without laparoscopy: a percutaneous endoscopic technique. J Pediatr Surg. 1980;15(6):872–5.
30. Kwon RS, Banerjee S, Desilets D, Diehl DL, Farraye FA, Kaul V, Mamula P, ASGE Technology Committee, et al. Enteral nutrition access device. Gastrointest Endosc. 2010;72(2):236–48. https://doi.org/10.1016/j.gie.2010.02.008.
31. Braegger C, Tamas D, Amil DJ, Corina H, Sanja K, Koletzko B, et al. Practical approach to pediatric enteral nutrition: a comment by the ESPGHAN committee on nutrition. J Pediatr Gastroenterol Nutr. 2010;51:110–22. https://doi.org/10.1097/MPG0b013e3181d336d2.
32. Moller P, Lindberg CG, Zilling T. Gastrostomy by various techniques: evaluation of indications, outcome, and complications. Scand J Gastroenterol. 1999;34(10):1050–4. https://doi.org/10.1080/003655299750025174.
33. Pisano G, Calo PG, Tatti A, Farris S, Erdas E, Licheri S, et al. Surgical gastrostomy when percutaneous endoscopic gastrostomy is not feasible: indications, results and comparison between the two procedures. Chir Ital. 2008;60(2):261–6.
34. Grilo A, Santos CA, Fonseca J. Percutaneous endoscopic gastrostomy for nutritional palliation of upper esophageal cancer unsuitable for esophageal stenting. Arq Gastroenterol. 2012;49(3):227–31.
35. Ansilmo CB, Junior VT, Lopes LR, Neto JDS, et al. Surgical gastrostomy: current indications and complications in a university hospital. Rev Col Bras Cir. 2013;40(6):458–62. https://doi.org/10.1590/S0100-69912013000600007.
36. Dranove JE. Focus on diagnosis: new technologies for the diagnosis of gastroesophageal reflux disease. Pediatr Rev. 2008;29:317–20. https://doi.org/10.1542/pir-29-9-317.
37. Randolph JG, Lilly JR, Anderson KD. Surgical treatment of gastroesophageal reflux in infants. Ann Surg. 1974;180(4):479–85.
38. Kultursay N. Gastro-esophageal reflux (GER) in preterms: current dilemmas and unresolved problems in diagnosis and treatment. Turk J Pediatr. 2012;54:561–9.
39. Colletti RB, Chritie DL, Orenstein SR. Statement of the North American Society for Pediatric Gastroenterology and Nutrition (NASPGN). Indications for pediatric esophageal pH monitoring. J Pediatr Gastroenterol Nutr. 1995;21:253–62.
40. Washington N, Spensley PJ, Smith CA, Parker M, Bush D, Jackson S, et al. Dual pH probe monitoring versus single pH probe monitoring in infants on milk feeds: the impact on diagnosis. Arch Dis Child. 1999;81:309–12. https://doi.org/10.1136/adc.81.4.309.
41. Yoo BG, Yang HK, Lee YJ, Byun SY, Kim HY, Park JH, et al. Fundoplications in neonates and infants with primary gastro-esophageal reflux. Pediatr Gastroenterol Hepatol Nutr. 2014;17(2):93–7. https://doi.org/10.5223/pghn.2014.17.2.93.
42. Czinn SJ, Blanchard S. Gastro-esophageal reflux disease in neonates and infants: when and how to treat. Pediatr Drugs. 2013;15(1):19–27. https://doi.org/10.1007/s40272-012-0004-2.
43. Castellani C, Huber-Zeyringer A, Bachmaier G, Saxena AK, Höllwarth ME. Proton pump inhibitors for reflux therapy in infants: effectiveness determined by impedance pH monitoring. Pediatr Surg Int. 2014;30:381–5. https://doi.org/10.1007/s00383-013-3458-6.
44. Pacilli M, Chowdhury MM, Pierro A. The surgical treatment of gastro-esophageal reflux in neonates and infants. Semin Pediatr Surg. 2005;14(1):34–41. https://doi.org/10.1053/j.sempedsurg.2004.10.023.
45. Srivastava R, Bevry JG, Hall M, Downey EC, O'Gorman M, Dean JM, et al. Reflux related hospital admissions after fundoplication in children with neurological impairment: retrospective cohort study. BMJ. 2009;339:b4411. https://doi.org/10.1136/bmj.b4411.

46. Dala Vicchia LK, Grosfeld JL, West KW, Rescorla FJ, Scherer LR, Engum SA. Reoperation after Nissen fundoplication in children with gastro-esophageal reflux: experience with 130 patients. Ann Surg. 1997;2226:315–21.

47. Kubiak R, Spitz L, Kiely EM, Drake D, Pierro A. Effectiveness of fundoplication in early infancy. J Pediatr Surg. 1999;34:295–9. https://doi.org/10.1016/S0022-3468(99)90194-X.

48. Justo RN, Gray PH. Fundoplication in preterm infants with gastro-esophageal reflux. J Pediatr Child Health. 1991;27:250–4. https://doi.org/10.1111/j.1440-1754.1991.tb00402.x.

49. Kubiak R, Bohm-Starrm E, Svcoboda D, Wessel LM. Comparison of long-term outcomes between open and laparoscopic Thal fundoplication in children. J Pediatr Surg. 2014;49:1069–74. https://doi.org/10.1016/j.jpedsurg.2014.02.077.

50. Jackson HT, Kane TD. Surgical management of pediatric gastroesophageal reflux disease. Res Pract. 2013;2013:863527. https://doi.org/10.1155/2013/863527.

51. Blair A, Jobe BA, John G, Hunter JG, David I, Watson DI. Esophagus and diaphragmatic hernia. In: Brunicardi FC, Billiar TR, Dunn DL, Hunter JG, Mathews JB, Polock RE, editors. Schwartz's principles of surgery. 9th ed. New York, NY: McGraw-Hill; 2010.

52. Snyder CL, Ramachandran V, Kennedy AP, Gittes GK, Ashcraft KW, Holder TM. Efficacy of partial wrap fundoplication for gastro-esophageal reflux after repair of esophageal atresia. J Pediatr Surg. 1997;32(7):1089. https://doi.org/10.1016/S0022-3468(97)90405-X089-1091.

53. Mayr J, Sauer H, Huber A, Pilhatsch A, Ratschek M. Modified Toupet wrap for gastro-esophageal reflux in childhood. Eur J Pediatr Surg. 1998;8(2):75–80. https://doi.org/10.105 5/s-2008-1071125.

54. Esposito C, Montupet P, van Der Zee D, Settimi A, Paye-Jaouen A, Centonze A, et al. Long term outcome of laparoscopic Nissen, Toupet, and Thal antireflux procedures for neurologically normal children with gastroesophageal reflux disease. Surg Endosc. 2006;20(6):855–8. https://doi.org/10.1007/s00464-005-0501-2.

55. Kubiak R, Andrews J, Grant HW. Long term outcome of laparoscopic Nissen fundoplication compared with laparoscopic Thal fundoplication in children: a prospective, randomized study. Ann Surg. 2000;35(8):1214–6. https://doi.org/10.1097/SLA.0b013e3181fc98a0.

56. Maxson RT, Harp S, Jackson RJ, Smith SD, Wagner CW. Delayed gastric emptying in neurologically impaired children with gastroesophageal reflux: the role of pyloroplasty. J Pediatr Surg. 1994;29(6):726–9.

57. Pacilli M, Pierro A, Lindley KJ, Curry JI, Eaton S. Gastric emptying is accelerated following laparoscopic Nissen fundoplication. Eur J Pediatr Surg. 2008;18(6):395–7. https://doi.org/10. 1055/s-2008-1038919.

58. Wilson GJP, van der Zee DC, Bax NMA. Endoscopic gastrostomy placement in the child with gastroesophageal reflux: is concomitant antireflux surgery indicated? J Pediatr Surg. 2006;41(8):1441–144. https://doi.org/10.1016/j.jpedsurg.2006.04.021.

59. Rothenberg SS. The first decade's experience with laparoscopic Nissen fundoplication in infants and children. J Pediatr Surg. 2005;40(1):142–7. https://doi.org/10.1016/j. jpedsurg.2004.09.031.

60. Kane TD, Brown MF, Chen MK. Position paper on laparoscopic antireflux operations in infants and children for gastroesophageal reflux disease. J Pediatr Surg. 2009;44(5):1034–40. https://doi.org/10.1016/j.jpedsurg.2009.01.050.

61. Capito C, Leclair MD, Piloquet H, Plattner V, Heloury Y, Podevin G. Long term outcome of laparoscopic Nissen-Rossetti fundoplication for neurologically impaired and normal children. Surg Endosc. 2008;22(4):875–80. https://doi.org/10.1007/s00464-007-9603-3.

62. Hunter G, Smith CD, Branum GD, Waring JP, Trus TL, Cornwell M, et al. Laparoscopic fundoplication failures: patterns of failure and response to fundoplication revision. Ann Surg. 1999;230(4):595–606.

63. Rothenberg SS. Laparoscopic redo Nissen fundoplication in infants and children. Surg Endosc. 2006;20(10):1518–20. https://doi.org/10.1007/s00464-005-0123-8.

64. Shariff F, Kiely E, Curry J, Drake D, Pierro A, Machoney M. Outcome after laparoscopic fundoplication children under one year. J Laparoendosc Adv Surg. 2010;20(7):661–4. https://doi.org/10.1089/lap.2010.0213.
65. Esposito C, Montupet P, Reinberg O. Laparoscopic surgery for gastroesophageal reflux disease during the first year of life. J Pediatr Surg. 2001;36(5):715–7. https://doi.org/10.1053/jpsu.2001.22943.
66. Cameron BH, Cochran WJ, Mcgill CW. The uncut Collis–Nissen fundoplication: results of 79 consecutively treated high risk children. J Pediatr Surg. 1997;32(6):887–91. https://doi.org/10.1016/S0022-3468(97)90643-6.
67. Bluestone CD, Kerry R, Sieber WK. Congenital esophageal stenosis. Laryngoscope. 1969;79:1095–101. https://doi.org/10.1288/00005537-196906000-00004.
68. Takamizawa S, Tsugawa C, Mouri N, Satoh S, Kanegawa K, Nishijima E, et al. Congenital esophageal stenosis: therapeutic strategy based on etiology. J Pediatr Surg. 2002;37:197–201. https://doi.org/10.1053/jpsu.2002.30254.
69. Jain V, Yadav DK, Sharma S, Jana M, Gupta DK. Management of long segment congenital esophageal stenosis: a novel technique. J Indian Assoc Pediatr Surg. 2016;21:150–2. https://doi.org/10.4103/0971-9261.182592.

Chapter 7
Anastomotic Stricture After EA Repair and Role of CES

Anastomotic stricture (AS) refers to the esophageal narrowing which leads to symptoms including dysphagia, FTT, aspiration, desaturation at feeding, and regurgitation [1]. There is no clinical picture that is specific or sensitive enough for its diagnosis [2]. Other complications including GERD, esophageal dysmotility, vocal cord malfunction, laryngeal clefts, Tracheomalacia and recurrent TEF might result in same clinical picture post-EA repair. Such complications might overlap AS and may coexist. Assessment of the degree of narrowing and its level in AS alongside other potential complications, which might be present simultaneously, is essential. Initial anastomotic narrowing as detected by esophagogram does not correlate with a symptomatic AS [3].

Diagnosis of Anastomotic Stricture

Investigations must be commenced if symptoms emerge to evaluate and diagnose the AS. Tools used in the diagnosis include contrast examination and endoscopy of the upper GIT. Contrast study would indicate esophageal morphology and might suspect related CES or additional anomalies. Endoscopy plays a crucial role in the diagnosis and treatment. Measurements for the AS are simple on static radiological images.

The Anastomotic Stricture Index (SI)

Said et al. [4] developed the index to determine the quantity of AS severity and track its subsequent reaction towards treatment. The $SI = (D - d)/D \times 100$ where D represents the esophagus diameters beneath the stricture and d is the diameter

© Springer Nature Switzerland AG 2019
A. Ibrahim, T. Al-Malki, *Congenital Esophageal Stenosis*,
https://doi.org/10.1007/978-3-030-10782-6_7

of the stricture. Even though the SI has already been utilized in some investigations to evaluate the AS level through endoscopic and radiographic measurements, its clinical impact and usefulness should be ascertained within larger sequence [2]. Dilatation is solely required if patients are symptomatic with SI exceeding 50%. In pediatrics, refractory strictures refer to SI having a remainder of over 10% following 5 sessions. A recurrent stricture implies recurrence of symptoms or the SI is more 50% following more than 1 month when SI of below 10% was attained [4].

The Esophageal Anastomotic Stricture Index (EASI)

Sun et al. suggested the Esophageal Anastomotic Stricture Index (EASI), as the AS severity and development predictor following EA repair [5]. In the past, there was no accurate prognostic tool for risk-stratifying patients following EA repair. The EASI refers to a tool within the post-operative analysis that will indicate positive and negative predictive values for developing clinically significant strictures. It will enable constructive comparisons of patient outcomes and treatments between institutions. It will enable parental counseling, patient follow up, and assist in locating at high-risk patients of stricture formation [5].

The EASI was produced from first esophagogram digital assessment (conducted 5–10 days following surgery). Ratios of two pouches were collected using the narrowest diameter of a stricture well-filled with contrast, divided by the maximal lower and upper pouch diameter for the lower (L-EASI) and upper (U-EASI). The average of lateral and antero-posterior projections was computed to obtain equal weight ratios on single L-EASI and U-EASI views as expressed in the equation below:

$$U - EASI : (\text{Lateral } d \, / \, D + \text{Anteroposterior } d \, / \, D) \, / \, 2$$

where d represents the diameter of the stricture diameter whereas D represents the diameter of the upper pouch)

$$L - EASI : (\text{Lateral } d \, / \, D + \text{Anteroposterior } d \, / \, D) \, / \, 2$$

where d represents the diameter of the stricture and D represents the diameter of the lower pouch.

A 0.25 ratio implies that anastomosis diameter is 25% of normal esophagus' diameter of the patient. The tighter the stricture, the smaller the ratio; Sun et al. posited that EASI constitutes an easy reproducible tool for identifying at-risk ASs patients, for guiding the frequency of follow-up visits alongside the scheduling for upper endoscopy or contrast studies, to relate the stricture severity with the efficacy of numerous treatment techniques, and undertake a comparison of anastomotic methods within patient registries [5]. Nevertheless, there is need for further studies to ascertain its reproducibility and usefulness.

Time for First Assessment of Suspected AS

Most surgeons would conduct the first esophagogram around 5–10 days postoperatively searching for complications including dysmotility, GER recurrent TEF, leakage and to discover associated anomalies such as CES. An anastomotic stricture found at that time is often regarded as a possible physiological stenosis as a normal process of healing and not a clinically appropriate stricture [3]. Early routine AS screening commences not prior to 21 days following EA repair to avert the risk for the anastomosis integrity. A closer look for a related CES is imperative. A scenario that was significantly suspicious of CES distal to the anastomotic region found in the first esophagogram, was reported. Our plan was to begin feeding with full antireflux measures and utilize the esophageal balloon after 21 days post operatively to confirm and dilate. Unfortunately, the condition progressed quickly to trigger serious brain damage due to pulmonary aspiration as illustrated in Fig. 4.3a–c.

Risk Factors for Anastomotic Stricture (AS)

In the majority of recent studies [2], it is reported that the incidence of AS after EA repair ranges from 32 to 59%.The risk factors leading to AS may be preoperative, intraoperative or postoperative. Preoperative risk factors include gap length, type of EA, gestational age, and associated malformation. Excessive mobilization of the lower esophageal pouch may affect its segmental blood supply and result in ischemia at the anastomotic site followed by stricture. A long gap is by far the most important predictive risk factor for early and late development of ASs. However, there is no agreement about the definition of a long gap. Intraoperative risk factors include degree of ischemia, anastomotic tension, and the type of suture material. There is an increased tendency towards reduction of delayed primary repair and esophageal replacement in favor of early primary repair [6]. This may result in anastomotic tension leading to AS. However, this can be decreased by care to include the mucosa in every suture of the anastomosis, preservation of the blood supply and meticulous handling of the esophageal ends. The Kimura advancement technique involves only the upper pouch. A multistage extra thoracic esophageal lengthening of the upper pouch by transferring the esophageal stoma step wisely further down the anterior chest wall. Foker technique includes aggressive mobilization of both lower and upper pouches outside the chest and progressively pulling them in the following days until it is possible to do the primary repair [7]. Further prospective studies for the evaluation and prevention of AS in such elongation techniques is required. A continuous suturing, two-layered or Haight anastomosis and end to side anastomosis are associated with increased incidence of AS and should be avoided.

Postoperative Risk Factors for AS

The risk factors for the formation of AS are leakage and gastroesophageal reflux disease (GERD). Leakage is more common with long gaps and predisposes to AS [8]. Excessive mobilization of the lower pouch with disruption of the GEJ may promote GERD. Acid reflux reaching to the anastomotic site facilitates AS as well as recurrent and refractory strictures. The ESPGHAN-NASPGHAN guidelines suggest a systematic routine treatment with proton pump inhibitors (PPI) for one year after surgical correction of EA even if evidence of the beneficial role of prophylactic PPI therapy is lacking [9].

CES as a Risk Factor for Anastomotic and Distal Esophageal Stricture

CES can affect the anastomotic site or distal to it and should be added to the risk factors of AS and non-anastomotic strictures [10, 11]. It is an important risk factor for recurrent and refractory strictures as well. If anastomotic histology shows TBR or FMD, or a CES distal to the anastomotic site is suspected, the scenario of AS and/ or dysmotility should be anticipated. A repeat barium swallow and meal should be done after 1 month of EA repair. Table 6.1 clearly shows that CES is a risk factor for refractory and recurrent AS.

Treatment of Anastomotic Stricture (AS)

The main line of treatment of esophageal stricture is conservative management with esophageal dilatation. Other adjuvant strategies for refractory and recurrent strictures may be required with dilatation. Surgery is reserved for extremely selected cases.

Prophylactic dilatation is not recommended [2]. Although there is no proof of the efficacy of routine H2 blockers or proton pump inhibitors (PPI) in preventing postoperative strictures, they are highly recommended [9]. Choking during feeding, intolerance to feeding, regurgitation, coughing, and apneic spells may be caused by anastomotic stricture. However, these symptoms may be due to other causes like GERD, recurrent TEF, tracheomalacia, swallowing incoordination, laryngeal cleft or CES at the anastomotic site or distal to it. These invite for esophagogram followed by tracheoscopy or esophagoscopy as needed. The initial esophagogram may show a varying degree of physiological stenosis during the normal healing process. So, we are left only with the clinical symptomatology to predict the development of stricture. This might be very late and significant morbidity or even mortality may occur especially for cases of CES. The EASI (see page 128) is a simple formulation (d/D), considering the upper and lower pouches independently. Sun et al. demonstrated that the lower pouch stricture ratio (L-EASI) is a superior prognostic test in determining the prognosis for an EA patient [5]. If the L-EASI is less than or equal to 0.30 is highly indicative for a course of dilatation. The family should be informed about AS and its risks and signs, and the necessity to repeat esophagogram if symptoms appear. Early diagnosis of the stricture increases the success and efficacy of dilatation before the development of fibrosis at 3–4 weeks after primary repair. Some would prefer to go for a diagnostic and therapeutic esophagoscopy and dilatation under general anesthesia (GA) instead of repeating esophagogram to avoid ionizing radiation. However, GA may affect neurocognitive development as well but early intervention is better to avoid protracted courses of dilatation under GA.

The EASI is an easy, reproducible tool to predict the development and severity of AS that can be used to identify patients at risk. It can guide the frequency of follow up visits and scheduling of esophagogram or endoscopy. It can be used in the future to correlate the severity of strictures with the efficacy of various treatment modalities and to compare different anastomotic techniques. The algorithm developed by Baird [1], has been modified to incorporate the EASI at initial esophagogram [5].

It is important to realize that stricture does not develop only in the anastomotic site after EA repair. CES can affect the anastomotic site or distal to it. A distal CES can be detected by failure to pass an NGT to the stomach during primary repair of EA or with a high index of suspicion in the initial esophagogram. The progress can be rapid and severe to cause morbidity or even mortality. Early diagnosis and dilatation by balloon might be of great help to avoid such complications.

In summary, the longer the gap length, the higher the tension placed on the primary anastomosis, resulting in GER and ischemia. There is also a risk of anastomotic leak, stricture and GER in cases of long gaps. An important unrecognized cause of post EA repair stricture is anastomotic or distal CES. Associated GER and dysmotility worsen the stricture and makes it refractory to treatment [10, 11]. Initial prophylaxis with H2 blockers is generally used. In high risk patients or those with an established stricture, proton pump inhibitors (PPI) become the prophylaxis of choice. However, recent evidence confirms that PPI alone do not necessarily prevent stricture formation. Patients who are refractory to anti reflux measures and dilatation may require a complete or partial fundoplication [12, 13]. For the last 12 years we are using partial anterior wrap as the preferred operation specially when there is esophageal dysmotility. Patients after Nissen fundoplication have a favorable outcome yet complications up to mortality were frequent after surgery [13].

Dilatation of Esophageal Stricture

The primary goal of esophageal dilatation is symptom relief, oral feeding without dysphagia and avoid pulmonary complications. Strictures due to caustic ingestion are complex (long segment, i.e. more than 2 cm and tortuous). Strictures secondary to EA repair are usually simple (focal, straight, large diameter). CES can cause stricture at the anastomotic site of EA or distal to it, the degree and severity of which cannot be predicted [10, 11].

Although bougies were the first tools to dilate esophageal stricture, balloon dilatation is now thought to be the safer and more effective except in cases of complex and severely fibrotic stricture where Savary dilators can be used. Current evidence supports the popularity of balloon dilatation over bougies [14].

Bougies are reusable and are more cost effective than balloons. They are of three types; those which are inserted blindly like Maloney are rarely used due to higher risk of perforation. Wire guided bougies like Savary-Gilliard are widely used. They have a long tapered tip and a radiopaque band at the beginning of the widest portion of the dilator to allow fluoroscopic guidance. These are passed over a guide wire, which is introduced beyond the stricture by endoscopy or under fluoroscopy (or both). Fluoroscopic guidance can be used during dilatation. Fixed-diameter bougie dilators exert radial forces and also cause a shearing effect with longitudinal forces during passage across the stenosis. Dilatation is considered done when there is a moderate or significant amount of resistance. The rule of three minimizes the risk of perforation. So, after a moderate resistance is encountered, no more than three dilators of progressively increasing diameters should be passed in a single session [15].

Balloons exert radial forces during dilatation. The force is delivered simultaneously over the entire length of the stenotic segment rather than progressively from its proximal to its distal extent. Through the scope (TTS) balloon dilator (Boston Scientific, Marlborough, MA, USA) are best done in children under general anesthesia with fluoroscopic or endoscopic guidance [11, 16]. In young children fluoroscopy is better used due to incompatibility of the TTS with small-caliber pediatric endoscopes. A special inflation system is required to adjust the balloon inflation pressure. Most authors use 1 min for balloon inflation, then deflation and reinflation up to three times in one session. Successful dilatation is detected by the obliteration of the "waist" under fluoroscopy. Most of publications wait at least 3 weeks after EA repair to avoid the risk of anastomotic disruption. There is no consensus regarding the interval between sessions. The interval ranges from weekly to monthly dilatation. However, most authors use a 2–week interval.

Bougie or Balloon Dilators

Complications of dilatation can occur even with the most experienced hands. Reported complications include, perforation, hemorrhage and bacteremia. Long term outcomes depend on the underlying pathology; stricture diameter and length.

Children with long gap EA postoperative anastomotic leakage and cases with associated CES are more prone to develop severe AS, which may be recurrent or refractory (Table 6.1). Currently, there are no randomized controlled trials comparing efficacy and safety of balloon dilator with bougie dilator for treatment of AS in children after EA repair. There were no significant differences between balloon and bougie dilators regarding safety and efficacy for benign esophageal strictures in controlled studies in adults. Therefore, the option to use bougies or balloons is solely premised on the operator's experience. The only suggestion of expert opinion from ESPGHAN-NASPGHAN involved the use of wire-guided dilators [9].

The necessity of repeating the dilatation is dependent on the stenosis diameter and length as well as the underlying pathology. Important risk factors include the presence of CES, GERD, and long gaps. The stricture in CES is usually complicated by recurrence coupled with the need of prolonged dilatation courses even following GERD control [11]. This applies for CES cases linked to EA rather than the isolated cases (Tables 6.1 and 7.1).

Table 7.1 Comparison between group A (CES associated with EA) and group B (isolated CES)

Criteria	Group A N = 16	Group B N = 11	P value
Sex			
Male	6	7	0.35
Female	10	4	
GA (weeks)			
Mean	35	36	0.62
Range	30–37	34–37	
Birth weight (kg)			
Mean	2.1	2.4	0.03
Range	1.7–2.9	1.9–2.8	
Age at first symptoms			
Mean	40.7 days	176 days	ᶜ0.001
Range	1–90 days	20–550 days	
Age at first dilatation			
Mean	49.3 days	20 months	ᶜ0.001
Range	1–60 days	1–60 months	
Associated anomalies	5 (31.3%)	4 (36%)	0.89
Types			
TBR (no cartilage)	4	0	0.09
TBR (with cartilage)	7	5	
FMD (by histology)	2	5	
FMD? (no histology)	3	1	
MD/FMD			

Site of CES (excluding 2 cases of pure EA with gastric pull-up)	Anastomotic
	  10 (71.4%)
	Distal to anastomosis
	  4 (28.6%)
	  2 whole LEP
		GEJ: 7
		Upper esophagus: 2
		Mid esophagus: 1
		Lower esophagus: 1	

The ESPGHAN-NASPGHAN suggests that no evidence exists to support the utilization of more invasive routine dilatation strategies; the AS must be treated solely among symptomatic children. A close-follow up is required in the initial 24 months of life, with the focus on the weaning stage. In long-gap EA patients, postoperative anastomotic leak require follow-ups and close observations to avert serious strictures. Based on experience, it could be inferred that CES cases linked to EA should be incorporated to the list.

Indwelling Esophageal Balloon for Benign Stricture

The balloon dilatation outcome is more preferable compared to bouginage with a success rate of 80–100%, with lesser number of dilatation (ranging between 1 and 40) required for curing stenosis for a period ranging between 2 and 42 months. The most prevalent complication is perforation (2–6%); however, in most instances, its treatment can be conservative. Some patients could be considered resistant towards dilatations, thus might need intra-esophageal stents. Stents do not lack complications including discomfort, obstruction, and dislodgement. Van der Zee et al. [17, 18] reported the utilization of indwelling balloon catheters in the treatment of resistant strictures. The authors investigated 19 children in 2014 and previously 2 cases in 2006. They alleged that using in-dwelling balloon catheters thrice per day dilatation has better tolerance among children and could easily be used by parents for self-dilatation at home. This helps maintain the optimal diameter of the esophagus. Keeping the child in lateral posture during balloon insufflations will not have any impact on the adjacent vena cava, aorta, or trachea.

A minor displacement risk exists. Marking on catheters would direct parents on correct catheter position prior to inflation. The perforation risk is negligible. A period of 4–6 weeks is appropriate for leaving balloon catheters in place. The main benefit of in-dwelling balloon catheters is that in entire day, the balloons are not insufflated enabling saliva and food passage. Additionally, it is hoped and believed that the technique could be used in CES cases as well as in esophagus caustic burns. The authors drew the conclusion that in-dwelling balloon catheters are safe and parents could use them at home. Notably, it removes the necessity for recurrent anesthesia, endoscopy, rethoracotomy and esophageal replacement.

Adjuncts to Dilatation

Steroids

When the strictures become refractory or recurrent after esophageal dilatation, a conservative method is still given preference through adjuvant treatments instead of opting for surgeries. Recurrent dilatation itself might induce intensive fibrogenesis in the process of healing. Recent evidence complementing the utilization of steroid injections for pediatric esophageal strictures are absent although it constitutes a recognized treatment in adults.

The real functional mechanism is not known. Steroid injection might decrease the synthesis of collagen and fibrosis. The most prevalent intralesional injection steroids include dexamethasone, betamethasone, and triamcinolone acetate. A 40 or 10 mg/mL, volume per injection in the range of 0.5–2.8 mL containing triamcinolone is administered using a standardized sclerotherapy syringe in 4 esophagus quadrants at the upper stricture borders prior to dilatation.

Studies on intralesional steroid injection safety and efficacy are heterogeneous, uncontrolled, and small. It is hard to draw definite conclusions concerning the benefits of intralesional steroid in decreasing repeated formation of stricture in patients with EA [9]. The ESGE-ESPGHAN requirements on pediatric gastrointestinal endoscopy are not supportive of the regular usage of intra-lesional steroid for refractory esophageal stenosis in children [19]. Similarly, there is no evidence to support systemic steroids in AS. However, evidence indicating that steroid injections alongside dilatation could decrease recurrent dysphagia risk within peptic-based refractory benign esophageal strictures. In contrast, addition of steroids to dilatation was ineffective within anastomotic stricture. The anastomotic stricture pathogenesis is different from that for peptic strictures; the pathogenesis in the latter is caused by acidic reflux ulceration and inflammation whereas in the former, it is caused by ischemia [20]. It is common belief that combining the two lesions is feasible and the steroids might be beneficial from this perspective.

Mitomycin C (MMC)

Mytomycin C (MMC) refers to a natural anti-tumor antibiotic, which reduces the formation of scars and fibroblast production. Local MMC application succeeded in decreasing the sessions of subsequent dilatation and modified symptoms in 75–80% of AS patients following EA repair. However, concern regarding gastric metaplasia at AS in 2 of the 6 patients in the short period of utilizing MMC existed [21]. Significant variability exists concerning the dosage (0.1–1.0 µg/mL), the application regimens ranges (1–12 applications) coupled with the administration route (antegrade or retrograde, without or with protective sheaths). One study did not find complications where 27 out of 31 patients exhibited excellent outcomes on short term follow ups [22]. The use of MMC must be targeted accurately to stenotic segments avoiding exposure towards adjacent healthy mucosa. The most common application method is localized application through cotton pledget dipped in MMC concoction in direct endoscopic observation [22].

Stricture spraying constitutes another potential method [23]. MMC must be newly prepared immediately prior to use. There was variation for the number of MMC applications from 1 to 12 alongside an average of 2 in children. The interval separating the applications was from 7 days to 13 months, alongside an average of 1 month [24]. Direct MMC injection into stenosis quadrant following dilatation has been cited in adults [25]. The most effective and widely used concentration is 0.4 mg/mL. Encouraging information on local MMC application are obtained from caustic refractory strictures [26].

Based on the ESPGHAN-NASPGHAN guidelines, despite contrasting existence of reports, MMC could be regarded as the possible adjuvant for managing recurrent strictures in patients with EA [9, 19].The evidence base of using MMC and steroids as a medical adjunct to dilatation is still weak. Nevertheless, both constitute reasonable first-line adjuncts in the event that dilatation does not succeed.

The Technique of Balloon Dilatation We Practice

To dilate or resect is a question which is almost answered [27]. Dilatation should be the initial management of all cases of CES even for the TBR type. The conservative treatment of esophageal stenosis and stricture rather than surgery is a well-known strategy for children. The esophageal morphology regarding stricture length, number and level and possible method of conservative management should be decided before treatment. The only target is normal food intake because there is no treatment that can resume a normal esophagus with normal motility at the level of the stricture. Our choice is the balloon dilator because of the radial force applied to the stricture and avoiding the axial force. It allows fluoroscopic visualization of the waist. The persistence of a portion of the waist means that the dilatation is only partially successful. Complete disappearance of the waist at the beginning of the first dilatation in a new session may be an end point for dilatation sessions.

Balloon dilatation under control of fluoroscopic guidance and general anesthesia with tracheal intubation is the preferred method in our institution. Significant esophageal stricture that requires balloon dilatation was diagnosed both clinically and radiologically. Intolerance to feeds, dysphagia and recurrent respiratory problems supported by esophagogram measurements are used to diagnose significant AS. We used to get the mean of the addition of the widest diameter of the upper pouch to the widest diameter of the lower pouch divided by 2. If the real measurement of the stenosis is 50% of the mean and the patient is symptomatic then this is an indication for dilatation. If it is 33.3% or less then it is a severe stricture otherwise it is mild to moderate. These measurements have been used long ago before other measurements [3, 4] came to light.

We did not usually do prophylactic dilatation routinely except in two conditions. The first is when the histology of the specimens at the anastomotic site collected during primary repair of the EA shows CES. The second is when the initial esophagogram is highly suggestive of a CES distal to the anastomotic site. At these two conditions, we observe the patients carefully and call for a repeat contrast study at the age of one month and a prophylactic balloon dilatation is indicated if there is a high suspicion.

The main indications for balloon dilatations are post- EA stricture, corrosive stricture, CES, peptic eosinophilic esophagitis and dystrophic recessive epidermolysis bullosa and others that will be mentioned later in details.

Repetitive esophageal balloon dilatation every two weeks with gradual step-up was used. Wire-guided, pressure-controlled multidiameter balloons (CRE, Boston Scientific Corporation, Massachusetts, USA) were used with fluoroscopic guidance. Flexible esophagoscopy was used only in difficult cases. The outcome was assessed by the response to the number of dilatation sessions, their effectiveness, and complications. A session is composed of three dilatations of 2 min duration each and 1 minute rest interval. The endpoint for dilatation was disappearance of the wasting at the first dilatation of the next session and then supported clinically. The response was considered excellent if one session of dilatation was required, satisfactory if up to five sessions were required and fair if more than 5 sessions were required. In case of GER with a stricture that does not respond to dilatations and full antireflux treatment, fundoplication and gastrostomy followed by dilatation are performed. In very difficult situations, with no evidence of a lumen simultaneous insertion of two guide wires one through the mouth and the other through the gastrostomy may be successful. In such difficult cases endoscopic guided wire insertion is tried. Delaying the procedure for few days may allow the saliva to trickle down through the stricture allowing the guide wire to pass.

The stricture was considered refractory if surgical resection was indicated due to failure of five dilatation sessions after fundoplication, or the stricture being too tight for a guide wire to pass. The dilatation was considered very effective if dysphagia disappeared, effective if it was still present to special types of food, or otherwise ineffective.

Patients younger than 6 months of age will respond better to dilatation [4, 28, 29]. Early detection and immediate balloon dilatation may prevent scar formation [30]. The time of early dilatation could be as early as 4 weeks after primary repair [29]. Dilatation which is done before 3 weeks could put the anastomosis at risk for perforation [31]. We performed a retrospective study in the pediatric surgery department of armed forces hospital, Khamis Mushait, southern region, Kingdom of Saudi Arabia in 2016 which was approved by the local Research Ethics Committee in the hospital (Tables 7.2 and 7.3) [11]. Eight patients were younger than 6 months at first dilatation in the non CES group. Four patients showed excellent response (one session of dilatation) while four showed satisfactory response (up to 5 sessions of dilatations). All ended up with a very effective dilatation (i.e. dysphagia disappeared). The total number of dilatations in the non CES group was 16 sessions (median = 1.5).

The CES group did not respect the above mentioned rules. Although all patients of the CES group were younger than 6 months when dilatation was initiated, three patients were refractory to dilatations. The total number of dilatation sessions in this group was 71 (median =3).

Table 7.2 CES group with anastomotic and distal stenosis

No./sex	Site of stricture	Degree	Risk factor	Treatment	Age (m)	Number of dilatations	Response to dilatation	Effectiveness / outcome
1. Female	Anastomotic	Severe	TBR/GERD/dysmotility	Dilatation/ARM[a]	2	5	Refractory	Ineffective
				Thal + GT[b]	4	–	–	–
				Dilatation	5	5	Refractory	Ineffective
				Resection	7	–	–	–
				Dilatation	8	6	fair	v. effective
				Dilatation	12	5	Satisfactory	v. effective
				Dilatation	24	3	Satisfactory	v. effective
				Dilatation	36	3	Satisfactory	v. effective
				Dilatation	60	3	Satisfactory	v. effective
2. Female	Anastomotic	Severe	TBR/GERD/dysmotility	Dilatation/ARM	2	5	Refractory	Ineffective
				Thal + GT	4	–	–	–
				Dilatation	5	5	Refractory	Ineffective
				Resection	7	–	–	–
				Dilatation	10	7	Fair	v. effective
				Dilatation	16	5	Satisfactory	v. effective
				Dilatation	24	4	Satisfactory	v. effective
				Dilatation	48	2	Satisfactory	v. effective
				Dilatation	72	2	Satisfactory	v. effective
				Dilatation	96	2	Satisfactory	v. effective

No./sex	Site of stricture	Degree	Risk factor	Treatment	Age (m)	Number of dilatations	Response to dilatation	Effectiveness / outcome
3. Male	Anastomotic	MM[c]	TBR/GERD/Major Dysmotility	ARM/Dilatation	1	1	Excellent	Ineffective
				Thal + GT + esophageal myectomy	1.5	–	–	Improved
4. Male	Distal	MM	? FMD GERD Dysmotility	ARM/Dilatation	1	3	Satisfactory	v. effective
				Dilatation	48	2	Satisfactory	v. effective
5. Male	Distal	Severe	Dysmotility/? TBR GERD/recurrent TEF	ARM/Thal/GT	1	–	–	–
				Dilatation	3	2	Refractory	Brain insult
				Esophagostomy	24	–	–	Mortality at 36 months
6. Female	Distal	Severe	GER Dysmotility FMD	Dilatation Dilatation/Myectomy Thal + GT	1	1	Excellent	v. effective

Ibrahim et al. [11]

[a]ARM = anti reflux measures

[b]GT = gastrostomy tube

[c]MM = mild to moderate stricture

Table 7.3 Non CES group with unremarkable histology and anastomotic stricture

No./sex	Degree	Risk factor	Treatment	Age (m)	Number of dilatations	Response to dilatation	Effectiveness of dilatation
1. Male	MM[a]	Long gap Minor leak	Dilatation	24	4	Satisfactory	v. effective
2. Female	Severe	–	Dilatation	1	1	Excellent	v. effective
3. Female	Severe	–	Dilatation	1	1	Excellent	v. effective
4. Female	Severe	–	Dilatation	1	3	Satisfactory	v. effective
5. Female	MM	Major leak	Dilatation	48	1	Excellent	v. effective
6. Female	MM	–	Dilatation	5	5	Satisfactory	v. effective
	Severe		Dilatation	24	2	Satisfactory	
7. Male	MM	GERD Recurrent TEF	ARM[b] Dilatation TEF ligation	3	1	Excellent	v. effective
8. Female	MM	–	Dilatation	3	2	Satisfactory	v. effective
9. Male	MM	–	dilatation	12	2	Satisfactory	v. effective
10. Female	Severe	Minor leak GERD	ARM/Dilatation	11	5	Satisfactory	v. effective
			Thal's fundoplication/ dilatation	18	1	Excellent	
11. Male	MM	GERD	ARM/Dilatation	5	2	Satisfactory	v. effective
			Thal's fundoplication	6	–	–	–
12. Male	MM	GERD	ARM/Thal's fundoplication dilatation	4	1	Excellent	v. effective
13. Female	MM	GERD	ARM/Thal's fundoplication/ dilatation	48	1	Excellent	v. effective

Ibrahim et al. [11]
[a]MM = mild to moderate stricture
[b]ARM = antireflux measures

Anastomotic Stricture in Non-CES Group has a Better Response and Effectiveness to Dilatation than CES Associated with EA

In the previous study a comparison was made between cases of stricture in EA and stricture in CES associated with EA in our institution. Table 6.1 shows significantly that the age in CES cases was younger at the start of dilatation, the number of dilatation sessions was greater, response to dilatation was worse as well as the effectiveness of dilatations. There were no refractory cases to dilatation in the EA group while there were 7/14 cases (50%) refractory cases in the CES group (Figs. 7.1 and 7.2).

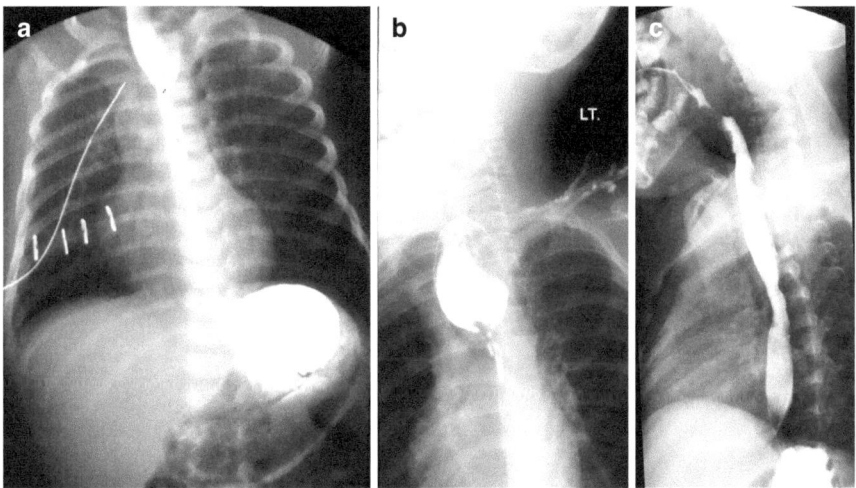

Fig. 7.1 (**a**) Initial anastomotic narrowing, no dilatation. If symptomatic or proved CES; dilatation to be done 3 weeks after primary surgery. (**b**) Severe anastomotic symptomatic stricture in a non-CES EA. (**c**) Successful balloon dilatation

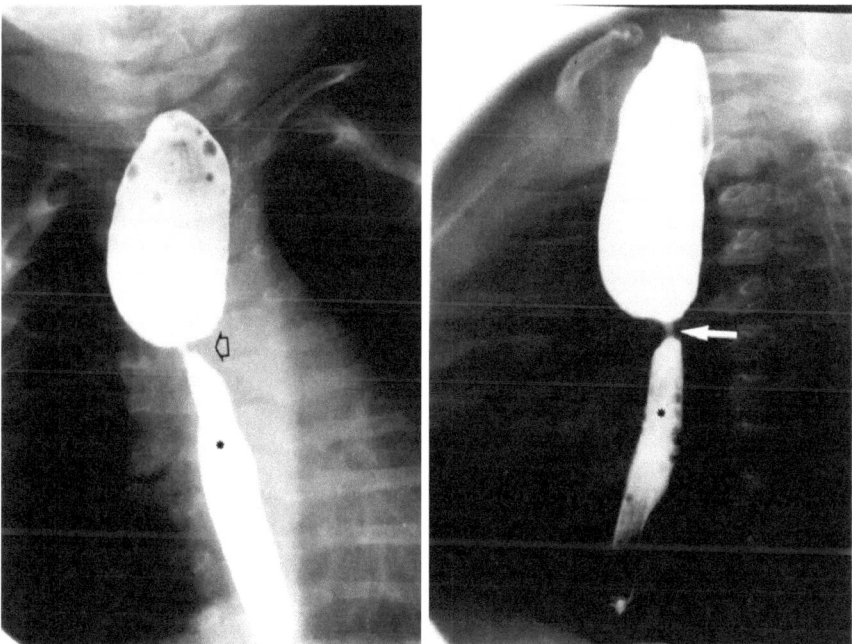

Fig. 7.2 Severe anastomotic stricture in two patients due to CES (TBR). Both showed failed initial dilatations with antireflux measures, both required Thal fundoplication, gastrostomy and dilatations followed by stricture resection then dilatation. Total number of sessions for each patient was 30 and 32 sessions respectively

The option of a more aggressive conservative strategies in the treatment of esophageal stricture with the goal of avoiding surgery and the goal to save the own patient's esophagus is a trial to avoid complications of replacement surgery. Intra-and postoperative complications may end up with anastomotic strictures, leakage, Severe GERD, bronchopulmonary disease, chronic dysphagia due to esophageal dysmotility and long-term low quality of life. Kasia et al. [32] reported their experience with 18 patients with CES over a period of 26 years managed by balloon dilatation as the only type of therapy offered. The mean *age* was 26 months with 80% of the patients above 6 months. Five patients (26%) had associated EA with distal fistula. Dysphagia was the main presenting symptom in 83% of the patients. CES was localized in the lower esophagus in 12 patients (67%), in the mid-esophagus in 3 patients (16%), and in the upper esophagus in 2 cases (11%). The site of CES was confirmed by endoscopy in 12 patients (66%) which also excluded peptic esophagitis. The number of dilatation was an average of two dilatations per child (range, 2–6 dilatations) over an average period of 6 months (range, 2–12 months). Esophageal perforation occurred in 12 balloon expansions (66%) all of which could be managed conservatively. The follow up was 11 years in average (range, 16–24 months). None of the patients required surgery and they remained asymptomatic with normal growth. The report mentioned above highlights that cases of CES can present late. There are different degrees of severity which cannot be predicted by the clinician. Incidence of perforation is really very high but fortunately could be managed conservatively.

Summary

Owing to higher rate of perforation and high number of dilatation sessions per patient, the treatment of strictures after EA surgery by bouginage was replaced by balloon dilatations. The rate of esophageal perforation with balloon dilatation is 0–10%, most of which can be treated conservatively. The best results are obtained when dilatation starts before 6 weeks before fibrosis develops but not before 3 weeks after EA repair. Associated GER worsens the results of dilatation mandating aggressive antireflux treatment and even antireflux surgery. GER is a significant factor in formation of refractory and resistant strictures. CES does not support the idea that early dilatation before 6 months will improve the dilatation results in cases of CES associated with EA. These cases have a worse response and effectiveness to dilatation. To minimize incidence of perforation, we use the proper sized balloons, avoid manipulation while the balloon is inflated. We also use water soluble contrast after dilatation for early detection of esophageal perforation.

References

1. Baird R, Laberge JM, Lévesque D. Anastomotic stricture after esophageal atresia repair: a critical review of recent literature. Eur J Pediatr Surg. 2013;23:204–13. https://doi.org/10.1055/s-0033-1347917.
2. Tambucci R, Angelino G, De Angelis P, Torroni F, Caldaro T, Balassone V, et al. Anastomotic stricture after esophageal atresia repair: incidence, investigation, and management includ-

ing treatment of refractory and recurrent stricture. Front Pediatr. 2017;5:120. https://doi.org/10.3389/fped.2017.00120.

3. Nambirajan L, Rintala RJ, Losty PD, Carty H, Lloyd DA. The value of early postoperative oesophagogram following repair of oesophageal atresia. Pediatr Surg Int. 1998;13(2-3):76–8.

4. Said M, Mekki M, Golli F, Hafsa C, Braham R, Braham R, et al. Balloon dilatation of anastomotic strictures secondary to surgical repair of esophageal atresia. Br J Radiol. 2003;76:26–31. https://doi.org/10.1259/bjr/64412147.

5. Sun LY-C, Laberge J-M, Yousef Y, Baird R. The esophageal anastomotic stricture index (EASI) for the management of esophageal atresia. J Pediatr Surg. 2015;50:107–10. https://doi.org/10.1016/j.jpedsurg.2014.10.008.

6. Orford J, Cass DT, Glasson MJ. Advances in the treatment of oesophageal atresia over three decades: the 1970s and the 1990s. Pediatr Surg Int. 2004;20:402–7. https://doi.org/10.1007/s00383-004-1163-1.

7. Sroka M, Wachowiak R, Losin M, Szlagatys-SidorKiewicz A, Landowski P, Czauderna P, et al. The Foker technique (FT) and Kimra advancement (KA) for the treatment of children with long-gap esophageal atresia (LGEA): lessons learned at two European centers. Eur J Pediatr Surg. 2013;23(1):3–7. https://doi.org/10.1055/s-0033-1333891.

8. Upadhyaya VD, Gangopadhyay AN, Gupta DK, Sharma SP, Kumar V, Pandey A, et al. Prognosis of congenital tracheoesophageal fistula with esophageal atresia on the basis of gap length. Pediatr Surg Int. 2007;23:767–71. https://doi.org/10.1007/s00383-007-1964-0.

9. Krishnan U, Mousa H, Dall' Oglio L, Homaira N, Rosen R, Faure C, et al. ESPGHAN-NASPGHAN Guidelines for the evaluation and treatment of gastrointestinal and nutritional complications in children with esophageal atresia-tracheoesophageal fistula. JPGN. 2016;63(5):550–70. https://doi.org/10.1097/MPG.0000000000001401.

10. Ibrahim AH, Al Malki TA, Hamza AF, Bahnasy AF. Congenital esophageal stenosis associated with esophageal atresia: new concepts. Pediatr Surg Int. 2007;23:533–7. https://doi.org/10.1007/s00383-007-1927-5.

11. Ibrahim AHM, Bazeed MF, Jamil S, Hamad HA, Abdel Raheem IM, Ashraf I. Management of congenital esophageal stenosis associated with esophageal atresia and its impact on postoperative esophageal stricture. Ann Pediatr Surg. 2016;12:36–4. https://doi.org/10.1097/01.XPS.0000482656.06000.84.

12. Snyder CL, Ramachandran V, Kennedy AP, Gittes CK, Ashcraft KW, Thomas M, et al. Efficacy of partial wrap fundoplication for gastroesophageal reflux after repair of esophageal atresia. J Pediatr Surg. 1997;32(7):1089–91. https://doi.org/10.1016/S0022-3468(97)90405-X.

13. Wheatley MI, Coran AG, Wesley JR. Efficacy of the Nissen fundoplication in the management of gastroesophageal reflux following esophageal atresia repair. J Pediatr Surg. 1993;28(1):53–5.

14. Al Shamrani J, Quesnel S, Pierrot S, Couloigner V. Endoscopic balloon dilatation of esophageal strictures in children. Int J Pediatr Otorhinolaryngol. 2011;75(11):1376–9. https://doi.org/10.1016/j.ijporl.2011.07.031.

15. Langdon DF. The rule of three in esophageal dilatation. Gastrointest Endosc. 1997;45:111. https://doi.org/10.1016/S0016-5107(97)70320-1.

16. Osuga T, Ikura Y, Hasegawa K, Hirano S. Use of endoscopic balloon dilatation for benign esophageal stenosis in children: our 11 year experience. Esophagus. 2018;15:47. https://doi.org/10.1007/s10388-017-0595-3.

17. Van der Zee DC, Bax NM, de Schryver JE, Beek FJ. Indwelling balloon dilatation for esophageal stenosis in infants. J Pediatr Gastroenterol Nutr. 2006;42:437–9.

18. Van der Zee D, Hulsker C. indwelling esophageal balloon catheter for benign esophageal stenosis in infants and children. Surg Endosc. 2014;28:1126. https://doi.org/10.1007/s00464-013-3288-6.

19. Tringali A, Thomson M, Dumonceau JM, Tavares M, Tabbers MM, Raoul Furlano R, et al. Pediatric gastrointestinal endoscopy: European Society for Paediatric Gastroenterology Hepatology and Nutrition and European Society of Gastrointestinal Endoscopy Guidelines. J Pediatr Gastroenterol Nutr. 2017;64:133–53. https://doi.org/10.1097/MPG00000000001408.

20. Ramage JI Jr, Rumalla A, Baron TH, Pochron NL, Zinsmeister AR, Murray JA, et al. A prospective, randomized, double-blind, placebo-controlled trial of endoscopic steroid injection therapy for recalcitrant esophageal peptic strictures. Am J Gastroenterol. 2005;10(11):2419–25. https://doi.org/10.1111/j.1572-0241.2005.00331.x.

21. Michaud L, Gottrand F. Anastomotic strictures: conservative treatment. J Pediatr Gastroenterol Nutr. 2011;52(Suppl 1):S18–9. https://doi.org/10.1097/MPG.0b013e3182105ad1.
22. Berger M, Ure B, Lacher M. Mitomycin C in the therapy of recurrent esophageal strictures: hype or hope? Eur J Pediatr Surg. 2012;22:109–16. https://doi.org/10.1055/s-0032-1311695.
23. Rosseneu S, Afzal N, Yerushalmi B, Ibarguen-Secchia E, Lewindon P, Cameron D, et al. Topical application of Mitomycin-C in esophageal strictures. J Pediatr Gastroenterol Nutr. 2007;44:336–41. https://doi.org/10.1097/MPG.0b013e31802c6e45.
24. Rustagi T, Aslanian HR, Laine L. Treatment of refractory gastrointestinal strictures with Mitomycin C: a systematic review. J Clin Gastroenterol. 2015;49:837–47. https://doi.org/10.1097/MCG.0000000000000295.
25. Machida H, Tominage K, Minamino H, Sugimori S, Okazaki H, Yamagami H, et al. Locoregional mitomycin C injection for esophageal stricture after endoscopic submucosal dissection. Endoscopy. 2012;44:622–5. https://doi.org/10.1055/s-0032-1306775.
26. El-Asmar KM, Hassan MA, Abdelkader HM, Hamza AF. Topical Mytomycin C application is effective in management of localized caustic esophageal stricture: a double-blinded, randomized, placebo-controlled trial. J Pediatr Surg. 2013;48:1621–7. https://doi.org/10.1016/j.jpedsurg.2013.04.014.
27. Koivusalo A, Turunen P, Rintala RJI. routine dilatation after repair of esophageal atresia with distal fistula better than dilatation when symptoms arise? Comparison of results of two European pediatric surgical centers. J Pediatr Surg. 2004;39:643–7. https://doi.org/10.1016/j.jpedsurg.2004.07.011.
28. Koivusalo A, Pakarinen MP, Rintala RJ. Anastomotic dilatation after repair of esophageal atresia with distal fistula. Comparison of results after routine versus selective dilatation. Dis Esophagus. 2009;22:190–4. https://doi.org/10.1111/j.1442-2050.2008.00902.x.
29. Antoniou D, Soutis M, Christopoulos-Geroula G. Anastomotic strictures following esophageal atresia repair: a 20-year experience with endoscopic balloon dilatation. J Pediatr Gastroenterol Nutr. 2010;51:464–7. https://doi.org/10.1097/MPG.0b013e3181d682ac.
30. Lang T, Hummer HP, Behrens R. Balloon dilatation is preferable to bougienage in children with esophageal atresia. Endoscopy. 2001;33:329–35. https://doi.org/10.1055/s-2001-13691.
31. Kim IO, Yeon KM, Kim WS, Park KW, Kim JH, Han MC. Perforation complicating balloon dilation of esophageal strictures in infants and children. Radiology. 1993;189:741–4. https://doi.org/10.1148/radiology.189.3.8234699.
32. Kasia A, Kechiche N, Mekki M, Nouri A. Balloon dilatation in congenital esophageal stenosis. J Neonatal Surg. 2017;6:90. https://doi.org/10.21699/jns.v6i4.647.

Chapter 8
What Should Be Done if Dilatations with Adjuncts Fail?

For recurrent and refractory strictures following adjunct-based dilatations failure, conservative management is still given preference at the expense of esophageal substitution. Esophageal replacement is characterized by a high morbidity risk, particularly in the long term. Refractory and recurrent strictures remain a major post-operative risk following esophageal substitution. Esophageal stenting and endoscopic electrocautery incisional therapy (EIT) might address the issue without requiring the heroic substitution surgery.

Endoscopic Electrocautery Incisional Therapy (EIT)

This functions by interrupting the fibrotic stricture tissues to obtain a suitable lumen diameter with needle-knife electrocautery. It involves numerous radial incisions parallel to the longitudinal esophagus aspect at the stricture region which is followed by balloon dilatation. Data on EIT efficacy and safety are mainly obtained from adults. Promising outcomes for AS and even in its capacity as the main therapy have been reported. Long strictures (over 1 cm) are characterized by worse outcomes with regard to recurrence.

EIT is safe and has minimal complications. There is scant data regarding EIT in pediatric population. The technique of endoscopic electrocautery has been practiced since 2002 [1]. Okada et al. reported three AS cases treated successfully following EA repair [2]. Nevertheless, there is scant evidence to propose it as the conventional AS treatment modality following EA. However, available evidence supports EIT use in AS among pediatric patients, particularly when the stricture is 1 cm or less [3].

© Springer Nature Switzerland AG 2019
A. Ibrahim, T. Al-Malki, *Congenital Esophageal Stenosis*,
https://doi.org/10.1007/978-3-030-10782-6_8

Esophageal Stents

In adults, esophageal stents were widely utilized. Stent usage in pediatrics was restricted because of inability of removing them if partial coverage or uncovered stents are used. Covered stents that are removable enabled its wide use in children and extended the directions for its use to feature various acquired and congenital esophageal strictures. Despite the absence of stents that are specifically designed for children, stents have been widely recognized in pediatrics for resistant stricture treatment, when endoscopic and medical treatments fail [4].Stents exert continuous and radially –driven pressure on esophageal wall for a prolonged duration, allowing the esophagus to retain patency through stricture stretching. This leads to remodeling of scar tissues and continuous luminal patency with decreased recurrent stricture development risks.

Three kinds of stents that are commonly used include biodegradable stents (BDSs), self-expandable plastic stents (SEPSs), and self-expandable metal stent (SEMs). The SEMs could be covered fully or partially by silicon or plastic membrane [5]. This enables the delayed removal of stents following a prolonged duration even though this could not be achieved totally in stents that are covered partially, an issue that reduced its application. Silicon membranes completely cover the SEPs, which have radiopaque markers placed at the ends and middle of the stents to facilitate their placement for fluoroscopy.

There is no need of removing the BDSs. They retain their radial distensile forces and integrity for around 6 weeks and disappear in 4 months following deployment [6]. The size of commercially available stents makes them unsuitable for use in children. However, biliary or airway stents might be utilized in pediatric population. Unlike esophageal stents, airway stents exist in various sizes but they are more rigid. Biliary stents have higher flexibility but only small sizes are available. To alleviate this issue that characterize biliary stents, custom dynamic stents designed from nasogastric tubes enclosed in silicon drainage tubes were used successfully [7].Various diameters and lengths are customized based on the level and size of the stricture. Its co-axial design on nasogastric tubes, guarantees it correct positions. Both ends are designed to permit easy introduction as well as passage of food between esophageal walls and the stent. Unlike other stents where passage of food is in the stents, the food within the dynamic stents passes between the esophageal wall and the stent, thus enabling long term esophageal patency improvement. Compared to the common metallic or plastic esophageal stents, the dynamic stent enhances esophageal motility compared to the common metallic or plastic esophageal stents [8]. Following dilatation, the customized stents are placed under fluoroscopic guidance. No suitable stenting period has been agreed upon yet. The duration ranges between 7 and 133 days in pediatrics, but 4–6 weeks may be ideal [9].

Caldaro et al. [8], conducted a research on 387 post-surgical EA correction patients from 1992–2012. The average age was 38.6 months (ranging from 3–125 months). Twenty-six of the three hundred eighty-seven patients were subjected to custom dynamic stent placement for recurrent strictures rather than serial dilatations. The stents were inserted following esophageal dilatations with the Savary-Gilliard dilators guided by fluoroscopy. All patients received 2 mg/kg/day of dexamethasone treatment for 72 h alongside 1–2 mg/kg/day lansoprazole or omeprazole (proton pump inhibitors). The stents were left intact for 1 month and 10 days and proved efficient in 80.7% (21 out of 26 patients). Two major complications related to stents, existed (subclavian-esophageal fistula). The author stated that dynamic stents are efficient and safe alternative in treating recurrent and severe post-surgical esophageal strictures. Surgery using resection and reanastomosis or jejunoplasty denotes the rescue surgery.

In another study that Foschia et al. conducted, [7], it was found that corrosive strictures are more refractory towards endoscopic therapy and required a significant number of procedures to achieve cure. Endoscopic corrosive stricture dilatations are more prone to complications compared to other stenotic forms. Therefore, in caustic stricture cases, the investigators opted to proceed by placing the stents directly to avert several complications of repeated dilatations. Additionally, they reported that stenting-related complications occurred less frequently compared to dilatation-related complications. Furthermore, stenting therapy decreased the time of treatment and averted recurrent anesthesia sessions required for dilatations. Hence, the stent denoted crucial improvements in therapies for benign esophageal stricture in children due to its tolerance by families and patients. They drew the conclusion that in caustic stricture patients, stenting denotes the initial option while in post-surgical strictures, the preference is on stenting only following a standardized dilatation program [10].

In contrast, Repici et al. [10] cited an experience of 15 years for refractory benign esophageal stricture (RBES) treatment in two academic facilities. They assessed the application of stents and dilatation for prolonged outcomes, resolution of adverse events, and dysphagia in 70 patients. Stricture resolution following an average follow-up duration of 43.9 months was attained in 31.4%. Success was less frequent in stent-treated patients (mean dysphagia -free duration of 72 days within the stent groups versus 99.5 days within the dilatation groups). The authors summarized that long-term outcomes for RBES treatment were disappointing, whereas stents did not have any additive impact on RBES' natural history. The strictures within the study were complex strictures as over 40% of the strictures were situated within the cervical esophagus where stent placement success is considerably low. Additionally, the length of the stricture was about 2 cm or longer. Therefore, the patients in the study had strictures that were significantly refractory.

Walter et al. [11] summarized their multicenter randomized research contrasting the placement of biodegradable stents with dilatations in 66 REBS patients. The main result was the endoscopic dilatation sessions number for recurrent dysphagia in follow-up. Besides, life quality and swallowing ability of patients that had received treatment were assessed regularly. Time towards the initial recurrent dysphagia episode necessitating interventions was considerably longer within the cohort featuring biodegradable stents than that for the dilatation cohort (median, 95 days against 30 days). Moreover, life quality was considerably better within the biodegradable stent groups than the dilatation group. Such outcomes prove that placement of stents must be taken into account as an important treatment option for RBES.

Future research should focus on developing novel biodegradable stents with maximum RBES management properties. Stents will have significantly high elasticity and radial force to decrease the stent migration and tissue in-growth risks; and with, a minimal axial force, to decrease serious adverse events as well as formation of fistula. Moreover, an integration of modalities that are currently available could be utilized together, for instance, esophageal stenting and electrocautery incisions [12]. A typical scenario constitutes the study that featured a novel method by Liu et al. [13], where the investigators utilized endoscopic incisions alongside esophageal stent placements for refractory benign esophageal stricture treatment. Only seven patients with the age ranging between 4 and 70 years featured in the study. Three patients had anastomotic strictures following EA repair, 2 following esophageal carcinoma whereas 2 were affected with caustic strictures. The stent was successfully removed 1–3 months following the procedure. Six of the seven patients (85%) showed an improvement in the follow up of 1–15 months following one treatment. The stricture diameter rose to around 1.0 cm–1.6 cm whereas the score of the dysphagia reduced to zero or one. One patient was diagnosed with a recurrence after 11 months of repeated incisions. One patient with stent migration required resetting. One patient had chest pain that healed after 5 days. The investigators concluded that using esophageal stenting and endoscopic incisions are effective, safe and feasible for RBES treatment.

Stents do not lack complications within pediatric patients. Migration to the stomach, stent displacement, and gagging have been cited. Life threatening events including granulation tissue, air way compression, and perforation, exist. Moreover, GERD and aspiration pneumonia have been reported. Stent erosion that causes arterioesophageal fistula is the major complication and it puts patients at the risk of mortality and severe bleeding [1, 12]. EA patients are characterized by higher occurrence of aortic arch and great vessels anomalies. This might put the patient at high risk of developing lethal complications. Esophageal stenting shows great promise as a tool for treating refractory and recurrent esophageal strictures. They are beneficial in sustaining luminal patency for prolonged durations and better feeding through the mouth. However, patient intolerance to stents coupled with the aforementioned complications are existing problems. There is need for prospective trials to document long-term safety and efficacy [3].

Custom dynamic stent implantation for post anastomotic (25 patients) as well as corrosive (55 patients) suffering from ES and high dexamethasone therapy dose (2 mg/kg/day for 72 h tapered for additional 144 h) was efficient in 88% of the patients [7, 8]. The investigators summarized that this kind of stent enables passage of food (an esophageal wall gym). The stent helps in the healing of strictures; at least, they help in shortening the strictures enabling anastomosis and surgical resection, averting esophageal substitution.

Metallic and plastic self-expanding stents were efficient in esophageal perforation patients [14]. They were efficient for treating post-anastomotic and post-dilatation perforations; however, they are inefficient in ES treatment with ES relapse occurring after the removal of the stents. Another study conducted in 2015 revealed that stenting denotes an effective and safe method for treating esophageal perforations [15].The conservative management of iatrogenic perforation subsequent to esophageal dilation constitutes broad spectrum intravenous antibiotics, nil per mouth and close checking for occurrence of any sign of mediastinitis with or without the aid of endotherapy. Endotherapy constitutes clip closure, endoscopic suturing and/or stent placement. Notably, usage of stents in pediatric population is only limited to post-operative leaks, refractory esophageal stricture, tracheoesophageal fistulas, and rare malignant conditions. Ahmad et al. [16] recorded an 18-month-old girl who had a congenital middle esophageal stenosis as a result of aberrant right subclavian artery. She a large esophageal perforation just after the esophageal dilation. The treatment was successfully administered to the patient by the use of a fully covered stent. The authors came to a conclusion that, with regards to selected cases, esophageal stent placement is much more feasible alternative to invasive surgery in iatrogenic esophageal perforation in children. Correspondingly, Rico ct al. [17] reported having employed a polyflex Airway Stent (Boston Scientific, Natick, MA) as an alternative treatment of esophageal stricture and perforation in an infant.

Rollins et al. [18], disclosed the initial case series report which talked about the usage of removable, covered stents for the treatment of persistent esophageal leaks. Three patients were notably reported to have esophageal perforation resistant to spontaneous non operative treatment and of which two of them had distal CES. More importantly to note, was the fact that all of the patients had a positive response to stent insertion. Arguably, it was regarded that persistent esophageal leaks should be treated by stenting because the covered stent will seal the perforation. This will allow patients to feed through the mouth.

The advice was to insert a stent if the esophageal leak failed to spontaneously seal after 2 weeks of aggressive nonoperative therapy. After stenting, intraoperative esophagogram is essentially carried out to confirm that no more leak is seen. The ideal stent posture is postoperatively confirmed by a chest radiograph. Endoscopy should be ideally done within a period of 1–2 weeks just after the administration of the stent to check for any esophageal erosion. The stent is taken off at a period of 3–4 weeks just after the placement is trailed by another esophagogram. While the stent is in place the proton pump inhibitors should continue and patient should be allowed to take any liquid food. However, if this is totally unachievable, then a nasogastric tube feeding through the stent is used.

Gebrail et al. [19], gave a full description of a full-term infant with severe and long esophageal stricture (5 cm × 4 mm) just after surgical correction of EA and TEF. The stricture was successfully dilated by the use of a biliary balloon dilator followed by the placement of a biliary stent that measured 10 mm × 6 cm for 6 weeks and the stent was removed. A fully covered esophageal stent that measured 12 mm × 70 mm was placed using a guidewire under fluoroscopic guidance and left for a period of 5 weeks. This yielded in a long period of patency and valfdness of the steps employed. Endoscopic biliary accessories followed by fully covered esophageal stents should perhaps be considered in postoperative severe esophageal benign stricture.

Lange et al. [15] disclosed the usage of a fully covered self-expandable stents made of metal ideal for benign esophageal stricture cases amongst children. Six boys and five girls were described having a median age of 30.5 months (range, 1 month–11 years) who were treated with SEMSs for benign esophageal condition. Four patients had esophageal stricture after EA repair, anastomotic leak in one, recurrent fistula in one and five had iatrogenic perforation. Notably, the stenting median duration was to be 29 days (range, 17–91 days). Four patients had four different SEMSs which were placed successively over time. There were no recorded complications during stent insertion or removal. It was noted that six patients representing 55% of patients required no further intervention, two patients who made an overall of 18% were in need of more than a session of dilatation. Three patients making up an overall of 27% lacked any improvements and were in need of definitive surgery. Minimal stent related complications were recorded in five patients who made up 45% of the patients. Therefore, in conclusion, the authors stated that SEMSs can be safe and effective only in selected cases in children.

Managing Complete Loss of the Patency of the Esophageal Lumen

In the instance that stenosis is so narrowed thereby leading lumen cannot be identified, an ERCP guide-wire can be used [20]. Once the lumen has been passed, the guidewire tip site should be identified under fluoroscopic guidance. A Savary dilator or an ERCP dilator is passed over the wire to dilate the stricture. The Rendez-vous method is also ideal and can be employed. This is due to the fact that it is a safe method which restores patency of the esophageal lumen in 80–100% of patients [21, 22] A flexible endoscope is passed orally to the esophagus until it reaches the level of obstruction. Another flexible endoscope is passed retrograde through the gastrostomy site upwards to the lower limit of the esophageal obstruction. The combination of the endoscopy and fluoroscopy determines the orientation of the lumen which is punctured by a retrograde guidewire. Hence, the lumen has a retrograde guide wire coming through the mouth and is essentially used for antegrade dilatation. Importantly, these very narrow lumens can function as a one-way valve. No excessive endoscopic insufflation to avoid massive gastric distension and gastric necrosis. The guide-wire should pass under endoscopic and real time fluoroscopic guidance as well [23].

The Refractory and the Recurrent Esophageal Stricture

Among several papers within the literature concerning benign, recurrent and refractory esophageal strictures, a uniform definition does not exist for guidance. It is cumbersome to determine the extent to which physicians have tried to ameliorate strictures within the papers. It is unclear whether to place refractory stricture definitions prior to or following other procedures besides traditional dilatations. Other possible related procedures may include Mitomycin, steroids, antireflux therapy, and fundoplication or stent placement.

Kochman et al. [24] suggested that recurrent and refractory strictures be considered anastomotic restriction due to fibrosis or cicatricial luminal compromise that leads to dysphagia clinical symptoms in the lack of inflammatory endoscopic evidence. This might exist due to the inability of successfully remediating the anastomotic narrowing to 14 mm in terms of diameter after five dilatation sessions at an interval of 2 weeks (refractory) or due to the inability of maintaining satisfactory luminal diameter for 1 month after the targeted diameter of 14 mm has been attained (recurrent).

The definition does not seek to incorporate inflammatory stricture patients or those having satisfactory diameter and dysphagia caused by neuromuscular dysfunction (for instance, post radiation and postoperative therapy). Groth et al. [23] defined refractory strictures as having several characteristics including 1-inability to attain required luminal diameter that allows solid food intake without dysphagia in spite of four recurrent dilatations at the interval of 15 days or 2-strictures, which necessitate surgical interventions at specific points. Prior to classification of strictures as refractory, it is imperative to ensure that proper treatment was given. While the strictures could be difficult to manage, a systematic and thoughtful method could enable good swallowing functions to be restored for the patients.

In fact there is no consensus about the definition of a refractory stricture or recurrent stricture. Patients who have a stricture whether due to CES, corrosive ingestion, post EA surgery or peptic stricture together with GERD, should control the reflux before five sessions of dilatations. Some may require an antireflux surgery for the stricture to have a better response to dilatation. In cases of severe forms of CES not involving the GEJ we observed that GER is common. This is associated with esophageal dysmotility and stenosis whether at the anastomotic site of EA or distal to it. This triad of stenosis, reflux and dysmotility carries a high risk factor for refractory and recurrent stenosis, morbidity and even mortality. The story starts with intolerance to feed, episodes of desaturation, aspiration or apnea episodes. If the previous histology at the anastomotic site shows CES, then we know that we are dealing of anastomotic stricture or a major esophageal dysmotility. Barium swallow will show the anastomotic stricture or stenosis distal to it. If there is associated GER, it should be treated with full antireflux measures together with a gastrostomy and repeat of dilatation sessions. Failure of dilatation (usually five sessions) means a refractory stricture that needs surgical resection and primary anastomosis. The resected specimen should be sent for frozen section biopsy to be sure that we are anastomosing a healthy tissue with normal histology. Post-operative dilatation may be required but obviously with a better response to dilatation. The major aim of this protocol of management is to save the native esophagus of the patient which is the best conduit in comparison to other procedures of esophageal replacement. In very difficult situations and before embarking to esophageal replacement other procedures should be tried like combined retrograde and antegrade dilatations (Rendez-vous procedure), indwelling balloon catheter (page), adjuncts to dilatations (steroid or Mitomycin), and esophageal stents.

Van Boeckel et al. [25] summarized the treatment selection of refractory benign esophageal strictures by an algorithm that is clear to follow. Dilatation with Savory or balloon remains the first step. Dilatation combined with intralesional injections with steroids can be considered for peptic stenosis, while incisional therapy is found to be effective for Schatzki rings and strictures less than 1 cm. After failure of these therapeutic options, stent placement can be considered. A final step includes self bouginage or surgery. Following this treatment algorithm means that most patients with a difficult to treat esophageal stricture can be managed without an invasive surgical procedure. Whether stent placement could be positioned at an earlier stage in the treatment algorithm is a matter of investigation in the future. The type of stent to be used best is also under investigation. The fully covered SEMS, the fully covered SEPS, the biodegradable stents and the customized dynamic stents need randomized trials to determine the optimal treatment strategy.

References

1. Baird R, Laberge JM, Lévesque D. Anastomotic stricture after esophageal atresia repair: a critical review of recent literature. Eur J Pediatr Surg. 2013;23:204–13. https://doi.org/10.1055/s-0033-1347917.
2. Okada A, Usui N, Inoue M, Kawahara H, Kawahara H, Kubota A, Imura K, et al. Esophageal atresia in Osaka: a review of 39 years' experience. J Pediatr Surg. 1997;32(11):1570–4. https://doi.org/10.1016/S0022-3468(97)90455-3.
3. Tambucci R, Angelino G, De Angelis P, Torroni F, Caldaro T, Balassone V, et al. Anastomotic stricture after esophageal atresia repair: incidence, investigation, and management including treatment of refractory and recurrent stricture. Front Pediatr. 2017;5:120. https://doi.org/10.3389/ped2017.00120.
4. Dall'Oglio L, Caldaro T, Foschia F, Faraci S, Federrici di Abriola G, Rea F, et al. Endoscopic management of esophageal stenosis in children: new and traditional treatments. World J Gastrointest Endosc. 2016;8(4):212–9. https://doi.org/10.4253/wjge.v8.i4.212.
5. Spaander MC, Maron TH, Fuccio L, Schumacher Escorsell A, Escorsell A, Juan-Carlos Garcia-Pagán JC, et al. Esophageal stenting for benign and malignant disease: European Society of Gastrointestinal Endoscopy (ESGE) clinical guideline. Endoscopy. 2016;48:939–48. https://doi.org/10.1055/s-0042-114210.
6. ASGE Technology Committee, Tokar JL, Banerjee S, Barth BA, Desilets DJ, Kaul V, Kethi SR, et al. Drug-eluting/biodegradable stents. Gastrointest Endosc. 2011;74:954–8. https://doi.org/10.1016/j.gie.2011.07.028.
7. Foschia F, De Angelis P, Torroni F, Romeo E, Caldaro T, di Abriola GF, Pane A, et al. Custom dynamic stent for esophageal strictures in children. J Pediatr Surg. 2011;46(5):848–53. https://doi.org/10.1016/j.jpedsurg.2011.02.014.
8. Caldaro T, Torroni F, De Angelis P, Foschia F, Rea F, Romeo E, et al. Dynamic esophageal stents. Dis Esophagus. 2013;26:388–91. https://doi.org/10.1111/dote.12048.
9. Karamer RE, Quiros JA. Esophageal stents for severe strictures in young children: experience, benefits, and risk. Curr Gastroenterol Rep. 2010;12:203–10. https://doi.org/10.1007/s11894-010-0105-4.

10. Repici A, Small AJ, Mendelson A, Jovani M, Correale L, Hassan C, et al. Natural history and management of refractory benign esophageal strictures. Endoscopy. 2016;84:222–8. https://doi.org/10.1016/j.gie.2016.01.053.
11. Walter D, Van den Berg MW, Hirdes MM. A randomized trial comparing biodegradable stent placement and endoscopic dilatation for recurrent benign esophageal strictures (Destiny study). United Eur Gastroenterol J. 2015;3(5 Suppl):A24.
12. Siersema PD. Treatment of refractory benign esophageal strictures: it is all about being "patient". Gastrointest Endosc. 2016;84(2):229–31. https://doi.org/10.1016/j.gie.2016.04.035.
13. Liu D, Tan Y, Wang Y, Zhang J, Zhou J, Duan T, et al. Endoscopic incision with esophageal stent placement for the treatment of benign esophageal strictures. Gastrointest Endosc. 2015;81:1036–40. https://doi.org/10.1016/j.gie.2014.10.037.
14. Manfredi MA, Jennings RW, Anjum MW, Hamilton TE, Smithers CJ, Lightdale JR. Externally removable stents in the treatment of benign recalcitrant strictures and esophageal perforations in pediatric patients with esophageal atresia. Gastrointest Endosc. 2014;80:246–52. https://doi.org/10.1016/j.gie.2014.01.033.
15. Lange B, Kubia R, Wessel LM, Kahler G. Use of fully covered self-expandable metal stents for benign esophageal disorders in children. J Laparoendosc Adv Surg Tech A. 2015;25:335–41. https://doi.org/10.1089/lap.2014.0203.
16. Ahmad A, Louis M, Song WK, Absah E. Esophageal stent placement as a therapeutic option for iatrogenic esophageal perforation in children. Avicenna J Med. 2016;6(2):51–3. https://doi.org/10.4103/2231-0770.179552.
17. Rico FR, Panzer AM, Kooros K, Rossi TM, Pegoli W Jr. Use of polyflex airway stent in the treatment of perorated esophageal stricture in an infant: a case report. J Pediatr Surg. 2007;42(7):E5–8. https://doi.org/10.1016/j.jpedsurg.2007.04.027.
18. Rollins MD, Barnhart DC. Treatment of persistent esophageal leaks in children with removable, covered stents. J Pediatr Surg. 2012;47:1843–7. https://doi.org/10.1016/j.jpedsurg.2012.05.001.
19. Gebrail R, Absah E. Successful use of esophageal stent to treat a postoperative esophageal stricture in a toddler. ACG Case Rep J. 2014;2(1):61–3. https://doi.org/10.14309/crj.2014.86.
20. Lew RJ, Kochman ML. A review of endoscopic methods of esophageal dilatation. J Clin Gastroenterol. 2002;35:117–26. https://doi.org/10.1097/0004836-200208000-001.
21. Baumgart DC, Veltzke-Schlieker W, Wiedenmann B, Hintze RE. Successful recanalization of a completely obliterated esophageal stricture by using an endoscopic rendezvous maneuver. Gastrointest Endosc. 2005;61(3):473–5. https://doi.org/10.1016/S0016-5107(04)02789-0.
22. Dellon ES, Cullen NR, Madanick RD, Buckmire RA, Grimm IS, Weissler MC, et al. Outcomes of a combined antegrade and retrograde approach for dilatation of radiation-induced esophageal strictures (with video). Gastrointest Endosc. 2010;71(7):1122–9. https://doi.org/10.1016/j.gie.2009.12.057.
23. Groth SS, Odell DD, Luketich JD. Esophageal strictures refractory to endoscopic dilatation. In: Pawlik TM, et al., editors. Gastrointestinal surgery. New York, NY: Springer; 2015. p. 13–22. https://doi.org/10.1007/978-1-4939-2223-9_2.
24. Kochman ML, McClave SA, Boyce HW. The refractory and the recurrent esophageal stricture: a definition. Gastrointest Endosc. 2005;62(3):474–5. https://doi.org/10.1016/j.gie.2005.04.050.
25. Van Boeckel PGA, Siersema PD. Refractory esophageal strictures: what to do when dilation fails. Curr Treat Options Gastroenterol. 2015;13:47–58. https://doi.org/10.1007/s11938-014-0043-6.

Chapter 9
Experience with Balloon Dilatation

Experience with Balloon Dilatation

We reviewed our experience of balloon dilatations over a period of 13 years (December 2002 to December 2015). Balloon dilatation was indicated for a variety of cases including cases of EA/TEF, CES, cardiac achalasia, cricopharyngeal achalasia and cases of corrosive stricture. Unfortunately we did not have the facilities for miniprobe endoscopic ultrasonography (MEUS) which is the only diagnostic tool that can provide an accurate evaluation of esophageal wall thickness and can differentiate CES subtypes [1–3]. That was a retrospective study performed in the pediatric surgery department of the armed forces hospital which was approved by the local Research Ethics Committee.

Dilatation for Cases of EA/TEF (Table 6.1)

The total number of cases studied was 126 cases of EA (with or without TEF). A total of 58 (46%) EA patients developed post-operative symptomatic anastomotic stricture requiring balloon dilatation (Fig. 7.1a–c). Four patients presented with foreign body impaction requiring endoscopic removal before dilatation. There were 32 males and 26 females. We divided the patients into two groups according to the onset of the stricture (onset of symptoms). The first group A are those who developed late stricture (2 years or older). This included 17 patients with a mean age of 5.8 years (range, 2–10 years). Group B are 41 patients with a mean age of 5.5 months (range, 1–18 months). All in all, the response was excellent in 37 patients (63.8%) (Who required only one session of dilatation). The response was satisfactory in 20 (34.5%) (Requiring up to five sessions). Only one patient had refractory response (required resection after five sessions of dilatations and had application of Mytomycin in extra two sessions). After seven sessions of failed

© Springer Nature Switzerland AG 2019
A. Ibrahim, T. Al-Malki, *Congenital Esophageal Stenosis*,
https://doi.org/10.1007/978-3-030-10782-6_9

dilatation, the patient had resection of the stricture and primary anastomosis. The patient had extra more four dilatations after resection after which the dilatation was effective. The dilatations were very effective in 57 patients (98.2%) (No dysphagia to any type of food) and only one who had resection, still with effective dilatation (has dysphagia to special types of food). The total number of sessions was 106 for all patients with an interval most commonly 2 weeks between sessions. There was no perforation in these two groups of patients.

Dilatation for CES Associated with EA (Table 6.1)

Sixteen patients had CES (11.1%). Five patients had FMD and 11 had TBR subtypes. Two patients with TBR of the whole lower pouches of pure EA were excluded from the study because the patients had gastric pull-up. Thirteen patients had symptomatic stenosis at the anastomotic site or distal to it requiring dilatations. One patient with TBR without cartilage did not have symptomatic stricture. Stenosis was diagnosed at a mean age of 49.3 days (range, 1–60 days). The response to dilatation was excellent (requiring one session of dilatation) in two patients (15.4%), Satisfactory (up to five sessions) in four patients (30.8%) and refractory (requiring resection) in seven (50%) patients. The dilatation was very effective (no feeding intolerance) in four (30.8%) patients, effective (intolerance to semisolid) in two patients (15.4%) and ineffective in seven patients (50%). The total number of dilatation sessions in all the 13 patients before and after surgical intervention for fundoplication and resection of the stenotic site was 106. There was an interval most commonly of 2 weeks between sessions. The problem of CES associated with EA is that it may need protracted courses of dilatation with prolonged periods of free intervals. We had four patients of this category with severe anastomotic stricture due to CES, but eventually they improved with a very effective dilatation after a range of 30–32 sessions of dilatations (Fig. 7.2). There was no perforation in this group of patients.

Table 6.1 shows clearly the great differences of the results of dilatation for the stenosis of regular non CES cases of EA with stricture in comparison with those with associated CES. The incidence of postoperative esophageal stenosis after EA surgery is more common in regular non CES cases than those with CES (46% vs 10.3% respectively). Patients of the regular non CES are older than those associated with CES (mean age 37.6 months vs 49.3 days respectively). The number of dilatation sessions required is much less than that required in the CES group (106 sessions for a number of 58 patients vs 106 sessions for only 13 patients of the CES group). The CES group definitely requires more protracted courses of dilatations than the non CES group to achieve a success point. Only one patient in the non CES group was refractory to dilatation in comparison to the CES group (1.7% vs 50% respectively). So, half of the patients in the CES were refractory to dilatation requiring surgical intervention. The dilatation in the non CES group was very effective with disappearance of dysphagia to all types of food in comparison to those of the

CES group (98.2% vs 30.8% respectively). The dilatation was ineffective in 50% of the patients in the group of CES requiring an alternative way of feeding like gastrostomy until surgical intervention for the stenosis.

Statistical Analysis

Statistical analysis of data was done by using SPSS 22 for IBM program. The data was described as mean [min/max] for quantitative data and numbers and percentage for qualitative data. Independent sample t-test was used to compare two groups in quantitative data and Chi-square test was used for qualitative data. P is considered significant if ≤ 0.05.

Dilatation for Isolated CES Involving the GEJ (Table 7.3)

We had 11 cases of isolated CES (not associated with EA). Seven cases were affecting the GEJ and four cases proximal to it. The seven cases at the GEJ were five males and two females. The mean age was 21 months (range, 1–60 months). The diagnosis was made depending on the clinical picture, esophagogram and esophagoscopy in older four of them. The esophagoscope showed the area of narrowing, normal mucosa and the scope could pass to the stomach in one of them but the scope could not pass in the other three patients. Balloon dilatation was the next step. Balloon dilatations failed in those four patients who had upper GI endoscopy. The first case was diagnosed as cardiac achalasia and treated by Heller's myotomy which failed to cure the patient. The patient was cured after resection of the stenotic area which histologically showed TBR. The other three cases had the same scenario but the scope could not pass the stenotic area to the stomach. This excluded cardiac achalasia and the diagnosis of TBR was confirmed intra-operatively by palpation and frozen section biopsy. The three patients were treated by resection and primary anastomosis. So, all of the four patients were resistant to initial 3–5 sessions of balloon dilatations and required resection and primary anastomosis.

The remaining three cases of the seven patients involving the GEJ had intolerance to feeds and recurrent respiratory problems. GI contrast study showed narrowing of the distal esophagus with dilatation of its upper part with esophageal body tertiary contractions and esophagoesophageal reflux due to distal obstruction (Fig. 9.1a, b). Since the patients were so young (1, 2, and 1 months) of age, the Upper GI endoscopy was not done and esophageal balloon dilatation was started. All the three patients were cured after two sessions of dilatations. FMD was highly suspected due to excellent response to dilatation with no recurrence at follow up for more than 3–4 years. One patient was complicated with GER which responded to conservative management. Histological specimens were not available. It is interesting to mention that one of the patients of the later group had a perforation after

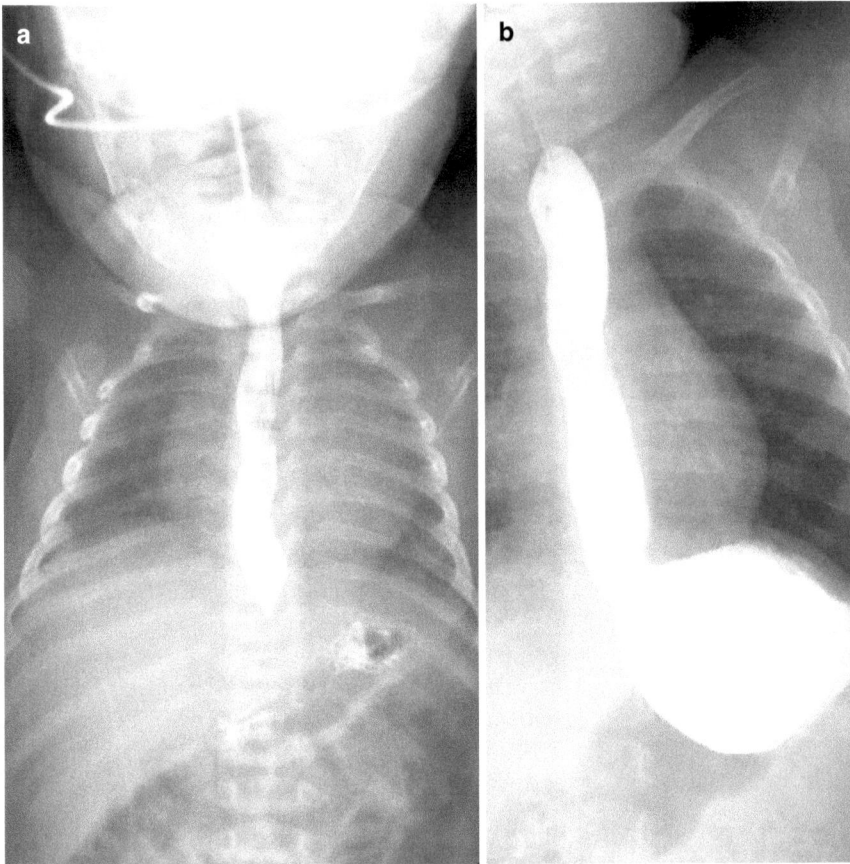

Fig. 9.1 A 21 days old girl with intolerance to feeds and recurrent chest problems. (**a**) Esophagogram showing cardiac achalasia like picture due to CES involving the GEJ. (**b**) esophagogram after successful three sessions of balloon dilatations

balloon dilatation as diagnosed clinically, X-ray abdomen and upper GI gastrografin study which showed leakage of the contrast from intra-abdominal esophagus. The abdomen was explored but the perforation could not be seen (sealed) and nothing more was done. The patient was cured with no recurrence of symptoms for 4 years follow up. We, presume that it was just a tiny perforation after balloon dilatation which sealed within hours.

Dilatations of Isolated CES Proximal to GEJ

Other cases of isolated CES not involving the GEJ were four cases in this review. The first case was a 4 year—old boy with Down syndrome who presented with a foreign body impaction in the mid esophagus. The foreign body was extracted and the stricture at the site of impaction as shown in esophagogram was dilated for three sessions the stricture was refractory to dilatation and required resection and primary anastomosis. The histology of the resected specimen showed TBR.

The second patient is a 3 months old female who was admitted to the pediatric ICU due to frequent vomiting and recurrent apnea. The upper GI contrast showed two areas of stenosis in the upper third of the esophagus (Fig. 4.1). Upper esophagoscopy showed a perforated diaphragm in the upper stenotic site. Bronchoscopy ruled out Laryngeal clefts or TEF. Balloon dilatation was performed for the two lesions altogether for three sessions. The patient was cured and remained symptom free for one year suggesting FMD. Of course, no histology specimen was available.

The third patient is an 18-month-old boy who presented in the NICU in the neonatal period with repeated desaturations, apnea and intolerance to feeds. An upper contrast study showed a thoracic stomach (Fig. 4.2a–c). That was repaired and a partial anterior wrap was also performed in the neonatal period. Few months later He was operated for VSD and ASD. At 18 months of age he was complaining of dysphagia to solids and semisolids. A contrast study showed a distal lower esophageal stenosis 4 cm proximal to the GEJ. An upper GI endoscopy showed normal mucosa and biopsy ruled out esophagitis. A late presenting CES was suspected and three sessions of esophageal balloon dilatation was performed. The patient was cured and remained symptom free for one year follow up.

The fourth patient was a 3 month-old girl who presented with recurrent desaturations, apnea and intolerance to feeds. Esophagogram showed a distal esophageal stenosis 3 cm above the GEJ. There was mild to moderate GER. Endoscopy showed a normal mucosa. Two sessions of balloon dilatation could cure the condition and the patient remained symptom free for one year follow up.

Balloon Dilatation for Cardiac Achalasia

We have only a little number of cases of cardiac achalasia. The reason is that most of the cases present after the age of 15 years. Our age limit as pediatric surgeons is only 14 years or less in our hospital. Also, most of the cases presenting in neonates, infants and young children are actually CES or peptic stricture rather than cardiac achalasia.

We dilated two cases of cardiac achalasia and three cases with cricopharyngeal achalasia.

The two cases of cardiac achalasia were a boy aged 11 years and one female aged 10 years. The boy complained of progressive dysphagia to solids and liquids for 3 years. There was weight loss as well. Barium swallow showed proximal esophageal dilatation, distal bird's beak appearance. There was aperistaltic esophageal body and there was no GER. There was a failure of the LES to open with swallowing; the contrast just trickled down to the stomach (Fig. 9.2a, b). Upper GI endoscopy showed a normal mucosa and the scope could pass easily to the stomach. This could easily rule out the possibility of peptic stricture. The differentiation between cardiac achalasia and a CES need to be confirmed. Five sessions of balloon dilatations were performed with only temporary relief of symptoms and the course was

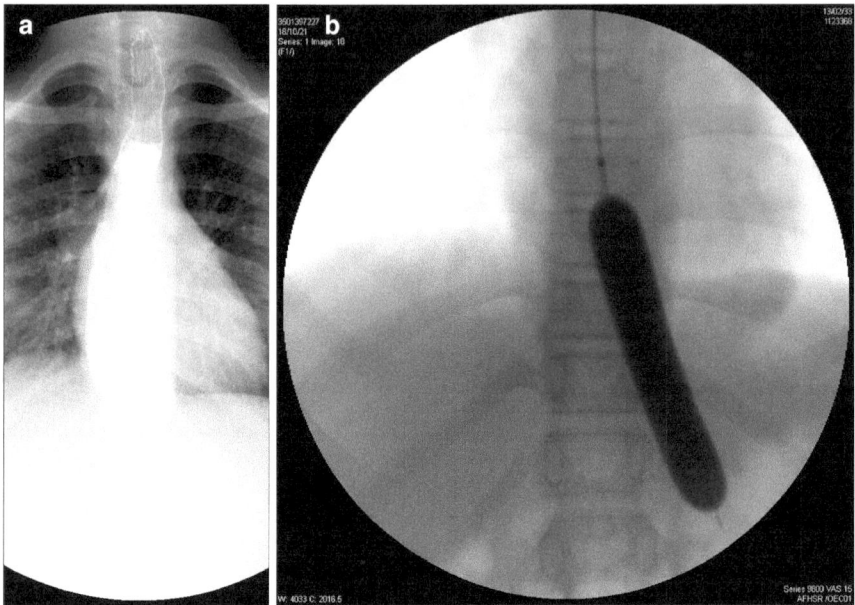

Fig. 9.2 An 11-year old boy with history of dysphagia for 3 years. (**a**) A dilated esophagus with typical bird's beak appearance suggestive of cardiac achalasia. (**b**) Five sessions of balloon dilatations gave only temporary relief. Lower esophageal myectomy and Thal fundoplication were successful. Histology showed no ganglia

progressive. The case was considered refractory to dilatation. Intraoperatively, there were no palpable ectopic nodules in the lower end of the esophagus. Myectomy instead of myotomy was done together with partial anterior wrap. The histology of the myectomy specimen showed absent ganglia confirming the diagnosis of cardiac achalasia.

The second case was a case of triple-A syndrome, an autosomal recessive disease characterized by the triad of adrenocorticotrophic hormone (ACTH) resistant adrenal insufficiency, achalasia and alacrima. This 10-year old girl used to come frequently to dilate her as a palliative treatment when severe dysphagia develops. This patient had three sessions of balloon dilatation, and then she was lost and did not come for follow up.

Dilatations for Cricopharyngeal Achalasia

A retrospective review was done over a period of ten years (December 2005 to Dec 2015).

We had four cases of primary cricopharyngeal achalasia with a mean age of 9 months (range, 7–10 months). The main complaints were choking, food regurgitation, nasal reflux, coughing, recurrent pneumonia, cyanosis and failure to thrive.

After ENT consultation, the diagnosis was confirmed with video fluoroscopy. Two patients were assigned as chronic lung disease (CLD) and massively refluxing patients requiring partial anterior fundoplication and temporary gastrostomy. Esophageal balloon dilatation was performed for all patients. One patient had excellent response after one session of dilatation. The other three patients required four sessions of dilatations for each patients. (Satisfactory response). The dilatations were very effective for all patients. Patients remained symptom-free for a period of follow up for 2 years.

Dilatation for Post Corrosive Stricture

A retrospective review was done over a period of 10 years (December 2005 to Dec 2015) for cases of post-corrosive stricture who required balloon dilatations. There were 13 patients with post corrosive stricture. There were eight females and five males. The mean age was 3.8 years (range, 1–6 years). Five patients had excellent response to a single session of dilatation. The dilatation was very effective and allowed eating everything. On the other hand, two patients had protracted courses of dilatation. The first patient had seven sessions of dilatation for the mid esophageal stricture. There was massive GER which might have affected the response with progression of dysphagia to semisolid food. A Thal fundoplication was performed together with a gastrostomy for feeding and for retrograde dilatations. Retrograde dilatations were performed for five sessions. Two more antegrade sessions using Mitomycin C (MMC) locally were performed after which the patient improved and the dilatations were very effective allowing feeding to all types of food. The gastrostomy was removed. Two years later, the patient had a foreign body impaction at the same site of previous stricture. The foreign body was removed and a single dilatation was performed. The patient remained symptom—free for 3 years.

The other patient had three sessions of dilatations but the effect was not encouraging. Barium swallow and meal showed massive reflux and a severe stricture. Thal's fundoplication together with a gastrostomy for retrograde dilatations and for feeding was done. The patient had seven sessions of retrograde dilatations followed by two antegrade dilatations with local Mitomycin C (MMC) applications. There was a dramatic improvement and the patient was able to eat all types of food. The patient is symptom—free for 2 years after the last dilatation.

Four patients with upper esophageal stricture improved after two sessions of dilatations and were able to feed normally. The remaining two patients were actually post battery ingestion stricture that required three sessions for each patient to be cured without further consequences.

Balloon dilatation (fluoroscopic guided) under general anesthesia is safe for a wide varieties of pathologies that required esophageal dilatation. We had experience with 305 sessions of dilatations with only two tiny perforations (0.65%) without mediastinitis that could be managed conservatively. Balloon esophageal dilatation under fluoroscopic guidance was introduced in 1981 by London et al. [5]. Since then it became popular for treatment of esophageal stricture because of its easiness and safety. The advantage of this technique is that the stenotic segment can be observed in detail under fluoroscopy, fluoroscopic monitoring during dilatation is possible, and the balloon–expanding force is exerted radially on the stenotic segment. Wire guided, pressure controlled with different sizes and diameters are available according to age and severity of the stricture. We did not use the endoscope to insert the guide wire except in very difficult strictures. Instead, we used the fluoroscopy to insert the wire which was quick and safe. We did not feel that it increases radiation exposure.

In summary, the use of balloons for dilatation of various benign esophageal strictures is safe and efficacious. It causes less damage to the stricture. However, Savary-Guillard bougies are more successful in cases of very rigid strictures. We recommend prolonged treatment of resistant stricture for CES and resistant strictures following burns.

Rupture is a rare complication of bouginage. This is less likely with balloons and it can be treated surgically with primary transverse suturing of the tear. When GER is present, it should be treated conservatively or surgically to sustain good results of dilatation. Dilatation should be the first line of treatment even in cases of TBR proved by Miniprobe EUS. Surgery should be reserved only for cases in which conservative treatment has been ineffective [6]. Surgery may end up with severe complications that lead to a recalcitrant stricture and a long-term low quality of life.

Stricture prophylactic key points for avoiding postsurgical ES were suggested by Groth et al. in 2015 [7] as follows:

1. For esophageal anastomosis: do an appropriately sized, tension free anastomosis and minimize risk factors for esophageal anastomotic strictures (e.g., ischemia and anastomotic leak)
2. For fundoplication and hiatal hernia repair: avoid doing a tight wrap and closing the hiatus tightly.
3. Use proton pump inhibitor for patients at risk for ongoing mucosal injury

Key Points for Managing Esophageal Strictures

1. Dilatation is the first-line treatment of esophageal stricture. Surgery should be reserved for failure of maximal nonoperative therapy.
2. Serial dilatations at 1–2 week interval may be needed to maximize the potential of dilatation and to achieve a satisfactory outcome.
3. Stenting is a temporary treatment option for benign strictures.
4. Rendez-vous procedure [8] is an excellent option for patients with complete loss of the patency of the esophageal lumen.
5. Always have a backup plan if the first choice of treatment fails or a complication happens

Diagnostic Challenges of Isolated CES Involving the GEJ

AS previously mentioned, Isolated CES cases involving the GEJ behave like cardiac achalasia and is usually misdiagnosed as such. They do not have GER and should be differentiated from achalasia and peptic stricture due to GERD [9, 10].

CES Wrongly Diagnosed as Cardiac Achalasia

CES due to TBR was first reported in 1936 by Frey and Duschel [11] in a 19-year-old girl who died with the diagnosis of achalasia. TBR diagnosis was established at autopsy.

In 1963, a full term baby had repair of EA and TEF on the first day of life. A size 5F transanastomotic tube passed to the stomach with some difficulty. There was a distended esophagus with air-fluid levels which required reexploration at 5 days of age. The distal 2 cm of the esophagus was narrowed and the esophagus above it was dilated up to the anastomosis. The esophagus was opened, dilated up to 8 F, closed and a gastrostomy was fashioned. Esophagogram after 2 weeks showed two anastomotic areas of leakage and distal esophageal stenosis presumed to be cardiac achalasia. Trials of dilatation up to the age of 5 months failed. A Heller's myotomy was done at the age of 6 months but the patient died after 10 days. Autopsy showed TBR at the level of the myotomy [12]. This report tells us that distal obstruction by CES can cause early anastomotic leakage (and similarly recurrent TEF) due to distal esophageal obstruction [13]. Also, early aspiration and recurrent pneumonia, all of which can lead to morbidity or even mortality. There are reports in the literature about recurrent TEF associated with EA together with CES. We learn also that a distal CES involving the GEJ mimics cardiac achalasia and the differentiation can be very difficult leading to errors in the management. A Heller's myotomy will not cure a distal CES with TBR involving the GEJ. In 1992, Yeung et al. [13] reported eight patients with CES due to TBR. With one exception, all were erroneously diagnosed as having peptic stricture due to GER in the distal esophagus. Nissen fundoplication was performed in three patients after failure of medical treatment and repeated dilatations. Patients did not improve except after resection of the stenotic esophagus. In 2000, Al Malki and Ibrahim [9] reported a 2 1/2-year-old girl complaining of persistent vomiting, severe dysphagia, recurrent chest infection and FTT. She was feeding only by a nasogastric tube. Chest X-ray showed areas of consolidation and bilateral bronchiectasis. Upper contrast study diagnosed the condition as cardiac achalasia. Esophagoscopy and biopsy was normal but the esophagus was hugely dilated and the scope could pass easily to the stomach confirming the diagnosis of cardiac achalasia. Manometry was not available. A trial of six consecutive esophageal dilatations failed. A Heller's myotomy did not help and the patient improved only after resection of the stenotic esophagus and primary anastomosis. Histopathology of the resected specimen showed TBR. Post-operative recovery was slow due to a hugely dilated esophagus. The patient was able to feed normally after one month. This is another example of an isolated CES due to TBR wrongly diagnosed as cardiac achalasia. An important lesson here is that the esophagoscope can easily pass the stenotic area even in cases of TBR with cartilage. Zhao et al. [14], considered a nonyielding esophageal stenosis without inflammation a characteristic esophagoscopic finding. They considered that the majority of cases of distal CES are diagnosed initially as cardiac achalasia or peptic stricture. They suggested that the esophagographic findings of TBR be classified into three types. Type Ia, the stenotic area is incompletely surrounded by cartilage presenting a tapered narrowing in the esophagogram. In type Ib the narrowing is radiologically abrupt due to a complete cartilaginous ring. In type II the ectopic TBR is very close to GEJ having a flask-shape shadow. Type III is either type I or II with linear projection of barium at the level of stenosis.

El Halaby et al. [10] reported 17 cases of CES. Fifteen patients were diagnosed primarily, while two patients were diagnosed after unsuccessful surgical treatment for an initial misdiagnosed achalasia of the cardia. They mentioned that in many instances it is difficult to differentiate CES from cardiac achalasia and secondary esophageal stenosis especially peptic stricture. One patient had a myotomy as a treatment for achalasia. The symptoms persisted after myotomy. Excision of the stenotic segment and colon interposition was required subsequently and the histopathology of the resected segment confirmed the presence of TBR.

In 2016, Kurian et al. [15] reported seven patients of CES. Six were in the lower esophagus and one was a mid-esophageal stenosis. Four patients were referred after trials of balloon dilatations. Two of them had esophageal myotomy for a wrongly diagnosed achalasia. They stated that clinical differentiation between CES, achalasia and GER related stricture is difficult. Barium study together with upper endoscopy and endoscopic ultrasound and MRI may be useful. An abrupt stenosis in esophagogram denotes TBR, whereas a tapered stenosis correlates with the FMD. This correlation of abrupt/tapered stenosis to the pathological type of CES might not be correct [16]. Endoscopy can diagnose reflux esophagitis and peptic stricture and the scope may not be able to pass the stricture. However, the mucosa is normal and the scope passes easily in achalasia. Endoscopic ultrasonography and MRI holds hope in the preoperative differentiation of TBR and non TBR types of CES.

Over a 14 year-period, we had seven cases with isolated CES involving the GEJ. Four cases had TBR which did not respond to repeated dilatations and required resection.

The remaining three cases were 20, 23, and 25 days old females with recurrent aspiration and intolerance to feeds. Esophagogram showed a picture like achalasia. Patients improved after three sessions of balloon dilatations for each.

Is it Cardiac Achalasia or CES?

Sir Thomas Willis first described cardiac achalasia in 1674 and the term achalasia was coined by Hurst in the year of 1927 [17]. It is a disease of adults because only less than 4% of all patients are symptomatic before the age of 15 years [18]. It is rarely seen in children and extremely rare in infants and neonates [17, 19, 20]. The etiology is not known. Esophageal body aperistalsis is due to absence of ganglia or degeneration of the myenteric plexus. The lower esophageal sphincter fails to relax with swallowing due to absent nitric oxide synthase which is responsible for synthesis of the neurotransmitter nitric oxide [21]. It is a progressive disease and the degeneration of intrinsic innervation of the esophagus gradually gets worth with age with symptoms becoming more obvious during adolescence and adult life. Congenital Chagas disease, as a cause of cardiac achalasia, is endemic in South America and can be excluded by specific tests. Detection of the living parasite T cruzi in the blood at any time after birth is diagnostic. Also, a positive T cruzi—specific serology in infants older than 8 months is diagnostic. A negative serological result in infants younger than 8 months of age rules out Chagas disease. Other possible medical causes for infantile achalasia can be primary abnormality of dorsal vagal nucleus as stated by Thomas in 1998 [22].

Only 31 cases of achalasia cardia in infants and only one report in a premature neonate had been documented in the literature up to 2016 [21]. We believe in the statement of Choudhury et al. that infantile cardiac achalasia have a different etiology [21]. The possible differential diagnosis of achalasia in young children, infants and neonates, are lower esophageal stricture due to GER and CES. The differentiation between cardiac achalasia, GER stricture and CES in neonates, infants and young children is essential.

Stricture Due to Gastroesophageal Reflux Disease (GERD)

Cases of cardiac achalasia and CES involving the GEJ do not reflux. GERD should be excluded by history, upper gastrointestinal contrast studies, flexible endoscopy with biopsy and specific pH/impedance studies if readily available. Stricture due to GERD is most unlikely in neonates and young infants. The history of GERD should be protracted in order to end up with reflux esophageal stricture which usually affects older infants and children. GERD in neonates and infants mainly present with respiratory problems rather than esophageal stricture. Barium swallow remains the most important tool to differentiate GERD from cardiac achalasia and CES affecting the GEJ in this young age. There is no GER in cases of cardiac achalasia or CES While reflux is readily seen and probably well-known from previous history and investigations in such a chronic patient. PH/impedance studies are of great help in cases of GERD. Upper GI endoscopy if feasible in very young neonates and infants will show mucosal changes like erythema, bleeding and ulcerations in cases of GERD. Biopsy will diagnose reflux esophagitis. The scope cannot be pushed down to the stomach in cases of reflux esophageal stricture. In achalasia the scope can pass easily to the stomach. The scope may or may not pass in cases of CES depending on the severity and type of CES [23]. TBR completely surrounding the stenotic area will not allow the scope to pass. Ectopic partial involvement may allow the scope to pass [9]. FMD cases with mild severity mostly will allow the scope to pass. The scope should be able to rule out an obstructing esophageal diaphragm. Kouchi et al. [24] reported a 7-month-old boy with frequent vomiting of milk with the esophagogram showing severe stenosis in the lower esophagus and esophageal dilatation proximally. Upper endoscopy identified a pinhole stenosis. EUS showed disruption of the submucosal layer and muscle propria layers at the stenosis with the 7-layered structures of the esophageal wall almost interrupted at the stenosis. The authors determined that the stenosis was caused by gastroesophageal reflux. The patient was treated by balloon dilatation followed by Nissen fundoplication.

Cardiac Achalasia in Neonates and Infancy and Young Children

Shettihalli et al. [20] reported that the incidence of achalasia is 0.5 to 1/100,000, with 3–5% of cases occurring in children and less than 0.5% in neonates. They reported the first case of achalasia cardia in a premature neonate. The baby had no prior symptoms and dilatation of the lower esophagus was incidentally discovered by chest X-ray. Esophagogram at 2 weeks of age showed cardiac achalasia. A nasogastric tube was inserted for feeding and another tube inserted in the esophagus for suction. A Heller's myotomy and fundoplication were performed at 36 weeks post conceptual age due recurrent aspiration. No endoscopy and no manometry and no trials of esophageal dilatations with good post-operative course at one year of age. In this case we do not know what excludes CES especially FMD subtype. Another term baby was reported at 2 weeks of age [19]. This case presented with repeated vomiting and aspiration pneumonia. A contrast esophagogram diagnosed cardiac achalasia and esophagomyotomy was performed at 3 months of age without any trials for esophageal dilatations. Again no endoscopy and no manometry and even no histology results available. Manometry will show specific finding of achalasia namely failure of relaxation of the lower esophageal sphincter with swallowing. Manometry is infrequently performed in neonates and young children due to its technical difficulties at that age and unavailability of suitable equipments. The diagnosis of achalasia cardia is likely to be questioned in these two cases simply because the diagnosis of the FMD type of CES cannot be ruled out and actually is more likely in this age.

Banerjee et al. [25] reported three cases of infantile achalasia cardia at 9, 7 and 12 months. The diagnosis was delayed because the cases were misdiagnosed initially as GER and treated for that without benefit. There was repeated non bilious vomiting, recurrent chest infection and failure to thrive. Cardiac achalasia was diagnosed by contrast swallow. No dilatation was tried and Heller's myotomy with fundoplication was curative. Similarly, Choudhury et al. in 2016 [21], reported a 6 months old infant with similar scenario. Chatterjee et al. in 2013 [17] published also two cases of infantile cardiac achalasia in 9 and 11 months girls. Regurgitation, chest infection and failure to thrive were the main features. Barium swallow diagnosed cardiac achalasia. Upper endoscopy was done to rule out congenital obstructive lesions. Modified Heller's myotomy with partial posterior fundoplication was curative. No manometry or histological results were available and no trials of dilatation were done. Consequently, CES of the FMD cannot be excluded. Esophagoscopy may be able to diagnose an obstructive diaphragm but cannot rule out other types of CES.

Krebit et al. in a letter to the editor [26] reported a female with history of desaturations since the neonatal period. At 2 months of age barium swallow was normal. At 8 months the barium swallow was repeated due to persistent vomiting and desaturations. The diagnosis of achalasia cardia was established. The patient was treated with esophageal balloon dilatations successfully. Again CES with FMD cannot be ruled out in this case. This type of CES usually responds well to esophageal balloon dilatations. Wong et al. [27] reported two cases of CES (TBR subtype) mistaken as cardiac achalasia. The first case was a 31-month-old boy with a two years history with repeated vomiting. Barium swallow was suggestive of cardiac achalasia. Upper GI endoscopy showed a normal mucosa and a tight stricture that did not allow the scope to pass. Dilatation failed and laparoscopic resection and primary anastomosis was done at 42 months of age. The histology of the resected specimen showed TBR. The second case was a 14-month-old girl who complained of repeated vomiting and loss of weight started at 6 months of age after introduction of solid food. Contrast esophagogram was suggestive of cardiac achalasia. Computed tomography showed a dilated proximal esophagus. The esophageal wall thickening at the stenosed segment was at the normal range. Endoscopy showed that the mucosa at the stenotic area was normal. The endoscope which was 5.2 mm could not pass. Balloon dilatation was ineffective. Laparoscopic resection of the stenosed area and primary anastomosis followed by Thal's fundoplication was performed. Histology of the resected specimen showed TBR.

There are examples of true CA in the literature. Starinsky et al. [28] reported a 10 months old boy with regurgitation and vomiting. Barium esophagogram showed a dilated esophagus with sluggish abnormal contractions. The lowest esophageal segment was narrowed allowing only small amount of barium to the stomach. The mucosa of the narrow segment was smooth and intact. Manometry studies of the esophagus showed tracings typical of achalasia. There was a high pressure zone of the lower esophagus with no relaxation during swallowing. The patient had a Heller's myotomy, Nissen fundoplication and temporary gastrostomy at 17 months of age after which the patient improved. A typical example of CA in children was given by Fernandez et al. [29]. They reported a case aged 9 months complaining of repeated non bilious vomiting and weight loss. Esophagogram showed a picture suggestive of CA. There was no GER and esophago-esophageal reflux was present with tertiary contractions, thus ruling out the possibility of GERD. Endoscopy encountered resistance at the cardiac end of the esophagus and biopsy showed chronic esophagitis with acanthosis. Manometry showed no relaxation of the LES with swallowing and increased basal pressure typical of CA. The patient improved after cardiomyectomy (instead of myotomy) and anterior partial wrap. The myectomy specimen showed neural threads and an absence of ganglion cells. That was a typical case of CA. Few years ago; we had a 9-year-old boy in our institution complaining of dysphagia and repeated vomiting. Contrast esophagogram showed achalasia-like picture (Fig. 9.2a, b). There was also tertiary esophageal contraction with very weak propulsive waves. Upper GI endoscopy showed the area of stenosis with normal mucosa. Biopsy was normal and the scope could pass easily to the stomach. Repeated balloon dilatation for five sessions offered only temporary relief and finally the condition got worse. Cardio esophageal myectomy was performed followed by a Thal's fundoplication. The histology of the myectomy specimen showed no ganglion cells. The patient improved and a follow up for 3 years was excellent.

Savino et al. reported a very important case for the dilemma of CES or achalasia in 2015 [30]. A term female baby with birth weight of 2810 gm was normal till the age of 6 months when weaning started. She started to refuse feeding, cry with gagging and vomiting. A diagnostic process was started by a tracheoscopy and neurological examination which were normal. Barium swallow was suggestive of cardiac achalasia. Esophagoscopy showed a normal mucosa and a tight stenosis that did not allow the scope to pass. Echoendoscopy (EUS) using a miniprobe showed regular thickening of the esophageal wall with no cartilage suggesting a FMD type of CES. The baby was cured after four sessions of balloon esophageal dilatation. If A Heller's myotomy was done, it would have been curative and the diagnosis is missed. If cartilage is present it would have not been curative and resection and primary anastomosis would have been required.

CES Involving the GEJ

This type of CES mimics cardiac achalasia. CES may be either TBR or FMD. The later type is not well appreciated in this location. The presentation may be early in the neonatal period or later when weaning starts. Mild forms of CES may be missed and present in the early years of life. The main symptoms are regurgitation, recurrent chest infections and FTT. This invites for a complete barium swallow and meal as the first step in the diagnostic process. Cooperation between the surgeon and the radiologist is essential. The study should look for the oral phase of swallowing, oropharyngeal disorder, cricopharyngeal achalasia, upper esophageal CES, N-type TEF, vascular rings, esophageal clearance, GER, hiatal hernia, gastric emptying and pyloric or duodenal pathology. In this situation the study will show a picture of cardiac achalasia. The 2nd step now in the diagnostic process is to differentiate between cardiac achalasia, stricture due to GER and CES as follows:-

- *Age*: The younger the age the more likely is the diagnosis of CES. Peptic stricture is unlikely in neonates, infants and young children. The history should be protracted to cause lower esophageal stricture. The patient will be very sick with very bad general condition. Cardiac achalasia is rare in young children, very rare in infants and extremely rare in neonates. It is worth mentioning that many of the reported cases of achalasia in infants might not be achalasia especially when proper investigatory tools were not used. CES can present in the neonatal period with variable severity [4]. However the symptoms may delay till the time of weaning when semisolid feeding start.

- *Contrast esophagogram*: the picture of achalasia with bird's peak appearance may dominate in the three conditions and it might be very difficult to differentiate achalasia from the other two conditions. However, if there is GER, then achalasia or CES are most unlikely. Aperistalsis of the esophageal body indicates achalasia rather than CES which may show vigorous contractions due to distal esophageal obstruction.

- *Upper GI endoscopy*: finding an inflamed mucosa with erythema, bleeding or ulceration is an indication of reflux esophageal stricture. Other investigations for GER like PH/Impedance technology are very helpful. The scope cannot pass the reflux stricture to the stomach. On the other side if the lower esophageal mucosa is normal and the scope cannot pass to the stomach, then CES is most likely. However, the scope may be able to pass in some cases of incomplete obstruction. In some cases biopsy from the esophagus may give a clue for CES although this is not usually the case because of the deep seated lesions. In achalasia cardia the mucosa is normal and the scope can pass easily to the stomach without difficulty.

- *Nasogastric tube (NGT) for feeding*: passage of NGT for feeding dramatically improves feeding and minimizes respiratory problems in cases of achalasia and CES but not so in cases of peptic stricture. Another tube in the esophagus for drainage of secretions avoids aspiration and its consequences. The problem of this drainage tube is the frequent dislodgment. It is possible that with this techniques we can buy time for those who are too young to have upper GI endoscopy and manometry. Also it gives time for the patient to be optimized for further management.

- *Manometry*: Although manometry is the gold standard in diagnosing achalasia cardia, many centers do not have this facility. It may not be possible to be done in young children and infants due to technical difficulties. There are several limitations for the use of conventional manometry in young children and infants. The catheter size and water perfusion rate in children differ from those in adults and need to be adjusted according to the age and size of the patient. The results of the manometry studies are difficult to interpret when there is crying or movement artifacts. The lack of studies in healthy children may also make the interpretation difficult and subjective [31]. *Four manometric findings are characteristic for cardiac achalasia*: (1) Increases LES resting pressure. (2) Incomplete or absent LES relaxation. (3) Absence of esophageal peristalsis. (4) Elevated intra esophageal pressure as compared with intra gastric pressure [32]. The high-resolution manometry (HRM) probably is going to replace the conventional manometry although the experience in children is limited. Kawahara in 2004 [33], reported the usefulness of video manometry in a case of CES due to TBR mimicking achalasia. Video fluoroscopy showed stasis of the contrast in the distal dilated esophagus associated with narrowing at the end of the esophagus mimicking achalasia. Manometry showed swallow-induced LES relaxation and low amplitude synchronous contractions in the whole esophageal body. Topographic plotting showed swallow induced LES relaxation and an absence of the second and third segments of the chain of sequential pressure events suggesting that the LES motor pattern is not compatible with esophageal achalasia.

• *Endoscopic Ultrasonography (EUS)*: The therapeutic plans for achalasia, CES due to TBR or FMD can be greatly different. Achalasia usually requires cardiomyotomy while most cases of FMD respond to dilatation. TBR requires resection anastomosis. Dilatation of stenosis due to TBR may end up by perforation [24]. So, preoperative distinction is essential. Miniprobe EUS with a maximum diameter of 2.5 mm has been useful in distinguishing such cases from each other [34]. The mini-catheter probe inserted via the working channel of the endoscopy is a safe and useful tool for evaluating high—grade stenotic lesions. Hyper echoic lesions will indicate TBR. If TBR is excluded then dilatation is the next step. If this fails after 3–5 sessions of dilatation then myotomy is indicated better with partial anterior or posterior fundoplication. However, if a TBR is diagnosed, a direct operation of resection and primary anastomosis is indicated without need for trials of balloon dilatations. LEE [34] reported a 12-year-old boy with history of vomiting dating since 5 months of age. Later there was history of foreign body stuck in the esophagus which was removed endoscopically. Later there was increasing dysphagia. Upper endoscopy showed the stenosis with no evidence of mucosal erosions. The scope could not pass down to the stomach. Esophagogram showed proximal dilatation and distal narrowing of the esophagus. Peristalsis of the esophagus was normal. All the above findings suggested CES and not achalasia. EUS showed multiple hyper echogenic spots into the muscle layer confirming TBR. Savino [30] reported a case of FMD involving the GEJ mimicking cardiac achalasia using EUS at the age of 9 months. The condition improved after four sessions of balloon dilatation.

• *Intraoperative differentiation*: When the upper endoscope passes the stenotic area to the stomach and the mucosa is normal, cardiac achalasia and CES cannot be differentiated. If dilatation is unsuccessful and EUS is not available, then intraoperative palpation for ectopic cartilaginous lesions can clinch the diagnosis. If still in doubt, we should go for frozen section biopsy. If TBR is confirmed resection and primary anastomosis with fundoplication is indicated. IF FMD or achalasia cannot be differentiated, we can perform myotomy and fundoplication. However, the authors believe that myectomy might be superior to myotomy because it allows a histological diagnosis if frozen section biopsy is not available.

Timed Barium Esophagogram

Timed barium esophagogram (TBE) is a simple and objective method for assessing the esophageal emptying. It is done by taking multiple sequential films at a pre-decided time interval after a single swallow of a fixed volume of a specific density barium solution. The volume of the barium suspension is usually 150–200 mL in adults and less than this in children as tolerated by the patient. Films are taken at 1,

2 and 5 min after barium. The degree of esophageal emptying can be assessed quali-tatively as well as quantitatively [35]. The height of the barium column is measured from its distinct superior level to the GEJ at the bird's beak appearance. The diam-eter of the esophagus is measured at the widest part of the barium column perpen-dicular to the long axis of the esophagus. Barium normally completely empties from esophagus in 1 min in most and 5 min in all healthy individuals. In cardiac achalasia there is esophageal aperistalsis with incomplete lower esophageal sphincter relax-ation leading to stasis and delayed emptying of the barium column. So, features of achalasia are delayed emptying of the barium column for more than 5 min, bird beak appearance of the LES, tertiary contractions of the body of the esophagus. This can be confirmed by manometry. The improvement of esophageal emptying after successful therapy (balloon dilatation or myotomy) can be more accurately evalu-ated by repeated TBE during follow-up using the same pre-treatment protocol. Less than 50% height reduction on the 5 min film in the post treatment barium column is considered a failure as per TBE. This is more likely in long standing achalasia with hugely dilated esophagus. Some studies have shown that TBE is as good as high resolution manometry to predict the response to balloon dilatation in achalasia patients [36].

Surgical Management of Unresponsive Stricture

Patients who fail to respond to all conservative measures will require a surgical inter-vention. A very little number of patients come to this point of surgical intervention [37].The most common procedure is resection of the stenosed segment and primary anastomosis. Despite of difficulty due to mediastinal adhesions the esophageal ends are in apposition with good blood supply hoping for success. Postoperative dilata-tion and even surgical revision may be required.

The decision to abandon the native esophagus and replace it is a major action. The reason is the significant short and long term associated morbidity after such major surgery. The esophagus may be replaced by a gastric transposition, colon interposition, jejunal interposition, and gastric tube. The choice between these tech-niques will depend on the individual and institutional expertise.

Surgical Resection

Patients with esophageal stricture who will require resection are fortunately small in number ranging from 3 to 7% [37]. Cases of TBR must be treated by surgical resec-tion either by resection of the stenotic region followed by end to end anastomosis or by enucleation of the cartilaginous remnants [38–41]. The resection can be done by open surgery. If the field is virgin, thoracoscopic or laparoscopic surgery is possible. After resection and end to end anastomosis, post operative dilatation is required again. This is more obvious in cases of TBR. Courses of redilatation sessions may be protracted and recurrence is the rule in CES [4, 42]. Interposition jejunal grafts, total esophageal replacement using gastric tubes, colon, or gastric transposition are exceedingly rare nowadays. The expected complications are anastomotic stricture, GERD, chronic respiratory problems, esophageal motility disorders and long-term low quality of life.

References

1. Teuri K, Saito T, Mitsunaga T, Nakata M, Yoshida H. Endoscopic management for congenital esophageal stenosis: a systematic review. World J Gastrointest Endosc. 2015;7(3):183–91. https://doi.org/10.4253/wjge.v7.i3.183.
2. Michaud L, Coutenier F, Podevin G, Bonnard A, Becmeur F, Naziha N, et al. Characteristics and management of congenital esophageal stenosis: findings from a multicenter study. Orphanet J Rare Dis. 2013;8:186–90. https://doi.org/10.1186/1750-1172-8-186.
3. Takamizawa S, Tsugawa C, Mouri N, Satoh S, Kanegawa K, Nishijima E, et al. Congenital esophageal stenosis: therapeutic strategy based on etiology. J Pediatr Surg. 2002;37:197–201. https://doi.org/10.1053/jpsu.2002.30254.
4. Ibrahim AHM, Bazeed MF, Jamil S, Hamad HA, Abdel Raheem IM, Ashraf I. Management of congenital esophageal stenosis associated with esophageal atresia and its impact on postoperative esophageal stricture. Ann Pediatr Surg. 2016;12:36–4. https://doi.org/10.1097/01.XPS.0000482656.06000.84.
5. London RL, Tortman BW, Di Marino AJ, Oleaga JA, Freiman DB, Ring EJ, et al. Dilatation of severe esophageal strictures by an inflatable balloon catheter. Gastroenterology. 1981;80:173–5.
6. Romeo E, Foschia F, de Angelis P, Caldaro T, di Abriola GF, Gambitta R, et al. Endoscopic management of congenital esophageal stenosis. J Pediatr Surg. 2011;46:838–41. https://doi.org/10.1016/j.jpedsurg.2011.02.010.
7. Groth SS, Odell DD, Luketich JD. Esophageal strictures refractory to endoscopic dilatation. In: Pawlik TM, et al., editors. Gastrointestinal surgery. New York, NY: Springer; 2015. p. 13–22. https://doi.org/10.1007/978-1-4939-2223-9_2.
8. Baumgart DC, Veltzke-Schlieker W, Wiedenmann B, Hintze RE. Successful recanalization of a completely obliterated esophageal stricture by using an endoscopic rendezvous maneuver. Gastrointest Endosc. 2005;61(3):473–5. https://doi.org/10.1016/S0016-5107(04)02789-0.
9. Al Malki TA, Ibrahim AHM. Isolated congenital esophageal stenosis: a case report and review of the literature. Ann Saudi Med. 2000;20:53–4.
10. El Halaby EA, El Barbary MM, Hashish AA, Kaddah SN, Hamza AF. Congenital esophageal stenosis: to dilate or to resect. Ann Pediatr Surg. 2006;2(1):2–9.
11. Frey EK. Duschel: cardiospasms. Ergeb Chir Orthop. 1936;29:637–716.
12. Neilson IR, Croitoru DP, Guttman FM, Youssef S, Laberge JM, et al. Distal congenital esophageal stenosis associated with esophageal atresia. J Pediatr Surg. 1991;26:478–82. https://doi.org/10.1016/0022-3468(91)90999-A.
13. Yeung CK, Spitz L, Brereton RJ, Kiely EM, Leak J. Congenital esophageal stenosis due to tracheobronchial remnants: a rare but important association with esophageal atresia. J Pediatr Surg. 1992;27:852–5. https://doi.org/10.1016/0022-3468(92)90382-H.
14. Zhao L-L, Hsieh W-S, Hsu W-M. Congenital esophageal stenosis owing to ectopic tracheobronchial remnants. J Pediatr Surg. 2004;39:1183–7. https://doi.org/10.1016/j.jpedsurg.2004.04.039.

15. Kurian JJ, Jehangir S, Varghese IT, Thomas RJ, Mathai J, Karl S. Clinical profile and management options of children with congenital esophageal stenosis: a single center experience. J Indian Assoc Pediatr Surg. 2016;21(3):106–9. https://doi.org/10.4103/0971-9261.182581.

16. Amae S, Nio M, Kamiyama T, Ishii T, Yoshida S, Hayashi Y, et al. Clinical characteristics and management of congenital esophageal stenosis: a report on 14 cases. J Pediatr Surg. 2003;38:565–70. https://doi.org/10.1053/jpsu.2003.50123.

17. Chatterjee S, Gajbhiiye V, De A, Nath S. Achalasia cardia in infants: reports of two cases. JIMA. 2012;44:44. https://doi.org/10.5915/44-1-9260.

18. Azizkhan RG, Taper D, Eraklis A. Achalasia in childhood: a 20-year experience. J Pediatr Surg. 1980;15:452–6.

19. Asch MJ, Liebman W, Lachman RS. Esophageal achalasia: diagnosis and cardiomyotomy in a newborn infant. J Pediatr Surg. 1974;9:911–2. https://doi.org/10.1016/S0022-3468(74)80229-0.

20. Chettihalli N, Veniogopalan V, Ives NK, Lakhoo K. Achalasia cardia in a premature infant. BMJ Case Rep. 2010;2010:1–4. https://doi.org/10.1136/bcr.05.2010.3014.

21. Choudhury KM, Begum T. Achalasia cardia in a 6-month-old boy: case report and review of literature. Birdem Med J. 2016;6(1):16–9. https://doi.org/10.3329/birdem.v6i1.28412.

22. Thomas RJ, Sen S, Zachariah N, Chacko J, Mammen KE. Achalasia cardia in infancy and childhood an Indian experience. J R Coll Surg Edinb. 1998;43:103–4.

23. Suzuhigashi M, Kaji T, Nogushi H, Muto M, Goto M, Mukai M, et al. Current characteristics and management of congenital esophageal stenosis: 40 consecutive cases from a multicenter study in the Kyushu area of Japan. Pediatr Surg Int. 2017;33:1035–40. https://doi.org/10.1007/s00383-017-4133-0.

24. Kouchi K, Yoshida H, Matsunage T, Ohtsuka Y, Nagatake E, Satoh Y, Terue K, Mitsunage T, et al. Endosonographic evaluation in two children with esophageal stenosis. J Pediatr Surg. 2002;37:934–6. https://doi.org/10.1053/jpsu.2002.32921.

25. Banerjee R, Prasad A, Kumar V, Wadhwa N. Infantile achalasia cardia. Indian Pediatr. 2016;53:831–2.

26. Krebit I, Murphy J, Awadalla S, Nicholson AJ. Frequent desaturations, vomiting and poor weight gain in an 8 month old. Ir Med J. 2012;105(9):314–5.

27. Wong HY, Chan KW, Lee KH. Congenital Esophageal stenosis due to tracheobronchial remnant: 2 cases report and literature review. J Paediatr. 2016;21:36–8.

28. Starinsky R, Berlovitz I, Mares AJ, Versano D, Pajewsky M, Modai D. Infantile achalasia. Pediatr Radiol. 1984;14:113–5. https://doi.org/10.1007/BF01625820.

29. Fernandez PM, Lucio LA, Pollachi F. Esophageal achalasia of unknown etiology in children. J Pediatr. 2004;80:5236. https://doi.org/10.1590/S0021-75572004000800016.

30. Savino F, Tarasco V, Viola S, Locatelli E, Sorrenti M, Barabino A. Congenital esophageal stenosis diagnosed in an infant at 9 month of age. Ital J Pediatr. 2015;41:72. https://doi.org/10.1186/s13052-015-0182.y.

31. Hong J. Clinical applications of gastrointestinal manometry in children. Pediatr Gastroenterol Hepatol Nutr. 2014;17(1):23–30. https://doi.org/10.5223/pghn.2014.17.1.23.

32. Tovar JA, Prieto G, Molina M, Arana J. Esophageal function in achalasia: preoperative and postoperative manometric studies. J Pediatr Surg. 1998;33:834–8. https://doi.org/10.1016/S0022-3468(98)90653-4.

33. Kawahara H, Kubota A, Okuyama H, Oue T, Tazuke Y, Okada A. The usefulness of video-manometry for studying pediatric esophageal motor disease. J Pediatr Surg. 2004;39:1754–7. https://doi.org/10.1016/j.jpedsurg.2004.08.032.

34. Lee KS. Diagnosis of congenital esophageal stenosis caused by tracheobronchial remnants using miniprobe endoscopic ultrasonography in a child. Pediatr Gastroenterol Hepatol Nutr. 2012;15(1):52–6. https://doi.org/10.5223/kjpgn.2012.15.1.52.

35. Neyaz Z, Gupta M, Goshal UC. How to perform and interpret timed barium esophagogram. J Neurogastroenterol. 2013;19(2):251–6. https://doi.org/10.5056/jnm.2013.19.2.251.

36. Goshal UC, Rangan M. A review of factors predicting outcome of pneumatic dilatation in patients with achalasia cardia. J Neurogastroenterol. 2011;17:9–13. https://doi.org/10.5056/jnm.2011.17.1.9.
37. Baird R, Laberge JM, Lévesque D. Anastomotic stricture after esophageal atresia repair: a critical review of recent literature. Eur J Pediatr Surg. 2013;23:204–13. https://doi.org/10.1055/s-0033-1347917.
38. Maeda K, Hisamatsu C, Hasegawa T, Tanaka H, Okita Y. Circular myectomy for the treatment of congenital esophageal stenosis owing to tracheobronchial remnants. J Pediatr Surg. 2004;39:1765–8. https://doi.org/10.1016/j.jpedsurg.2004.08.016.
39. Saito T, Ise K, Kawahara Y, Yamashita M, Shimizu H, Suzuki H, Gotoh M. Congenital esophageal stenosis because of tracheobronchial remnants and treated by circular myectomy. J Pediatr Surg. 2008;43:583–5. https://doi.org/10.1016/j.jpedsurg.2007.11.017.
40. Martinez-Ferro M, Rubio M, Piaggio L, Laje P. Thoracoscopic approach for congenital esophageal stenosis. J Pediatr Surg. 2006;41:E5–7. https://doi.org/10.1016/j.jpedsurg.2006.06.022.
41. Deshpande AV, Shun A. Laparoscopic treatment of congenital esophageal stenosis due to tracheobronchial remnants in a child. J Laparoendosc Adv Surg. 2009;19:107–9. https://doi.org/10.1089/lap.2008.0070.
42. Ibrahim AH, Al Malki TA, Hamza AF, Bahnasy AF. Congenital esophageal stenosis associated with esophageal atresia: new concepts. Pediatr Surg Int. 2007;23:533–7. https://doi.org/10.1007/s00383-007-1927-5.

Chapter 10
Congenital Membranous Disease of the Esophagus (MD)

This is also referred to in the literature as congenital esophageal web or diaphragm. This anomaly is actually the rarest of all types of CES.

Types of MD

The Non-Perforated Type of MD

This is an intraluminal completely obstructing type of the esophagus which present in the neonatal period with symptoms and signs of EA. There may be history of polyhydramnios, excessive salivation, chocking, cyanosis and inability to feed the baby. A nasogastric tube cannot be passed to the stomach which can be confirmed by an x-ray chest and abdomen. There are two types of this anomaly; isolated MD or associated with EA.

Isolated Type of Nonperforated MD

This is a congenital intraluminal mucosal web of the esophagus which is a very rare type of esophageal atresia. The etiology is not well understood. In this anomaly, the external esophageal appearance is normal upon surgical exploration. Only a few reports are available [1–6]. There may be a history of polyhydramnios, respiratory distress, failure to feed or passing an NGT. X ray chest and abdomen will show the NGT coiled at the site of obstruction together with a gasless abdomen. The site of obstruction is in the middle or distal esophagus. Esophagogram and esophagoscopy confirm the diagnosis. The treatment is by either surgical excision or endoscopic perforation and dilatation [6]. Patency of the distal bowel should be confirmed since an associated pyloric obstruction has been reported [3]. The histology shows squamous cell epithelium and connective areolar tissue.

© Springer Nature Switzerland AG 2019   133
A. Ibrahim, T. Al-Malki, *Congenital Esophageal Stenosis*,
https://doi.org/10.1007/978-3-030-10782-6_10

Nonperforated MD Associated with EA and/or TEF

These cases may be associated with VACTRL anomalies (*V*ertebral, *A*norectal, *C*ardiac, *T*racheoesophageal, *R*enal and *L*imb anomalies). They may present with history of polyhydramnios. They have symptoms and signs of EA and Chest X Ray and abdomen show coiled NGT in the upper pouch and gasless abdomen. Echocardiogram and abdominal USG should be done. The condition is usually discovered during primary repair of the EA/TEF. It is always mandatory to pass a NGT before completing the esophageal anastomosis. The distal esophageal obstruction is discovered and web excised through a small vertical esophagostomy. The web is reported associated with EA/TEF in the distal esophagus [7], and with isolated TEF at the level of carina in the distal esophageal pouch [8]. Also it has been reported that a complete obstructing MD was associated with isolated TEF having CES (FMD) in the mid esophagus and the web in the distal esophagus [9].

Congenital Perforated MD of the Esophagus

These rare anomalies are usually seen beyond the neonatal period specifically when starting solid food. There is dysphagia to solids, food and foreign body impaction [10, 11]. The main diagnostic tools are esophagogram and fiberoptic-esophagoscopy. The rigid esophagoscope may fail to diagnose the web [10]. Esophagogram shows a single thin indentation of the esophageal lumen that is located either anterior or circumferential in nature [12]. The web may be located in the upper third of the esophagus [12], mid esophagus [10] or distal esophagus [11].

Various methods have been used to treat the congenital esophageal perforated web. Dilatation alone using bouginage or balloons may be successful [10]. If balloon dilatation is not successful, then endoscopic electrocauterizaion with the aid of balloon dilatation can be used [11]. Roy et al. reported the first successful endoscopic laser division of the web in whom dilatation has failed [13]. Resection and primary anastomosis are rarely required.

References

1. Nanni L, Vallsciani S, Perrelli L. Congenital esophageal obstruction caused by mucous membrane: a clinical case. Cir Pediatr. 2001;14:38–40.
2. Sharma AK, Sharma KK, Sharma CS, Chandra S, Udawat M. Congenital esophageal obstruction by intraluminal mucosal diaphragm. J Pediatr Surg. 1991;26:213–5. https://doi.org/10.1016/0022-3468(91)90914 F.
3. Chuang JH, Chen MJ. Membranous atresia of esophagus associated with pyloric stenosis. J Pediatr Surg. 1987;22:988–90. https://doi.org/10.1016/S0022-3468(87)80489-X.
4. Abel AL. Congenital esophageal obstruction. Br Med J. 1928;2:46–9.

5. Pai GK, Pai PK, Kini AU, Rao J. Membranous type of esophageal atresia at the cardiac end of the esophagus: a case report. J Pediatr Surg. 1987;22:986–7. https://doi.org/10.1016/S0022-3468(87)80488-8.

6. Uguralp S, Ceran C, Demircan M. Congenital distal esophageal obstruction caused by intraluminal mucosal web. Turk J Pediatr. 2012;54:317–9.

7. Jaycar RD, Ubale BP, Agrwal SG. Tracheo-esophageal fistula with distal esophageal web: a case report. Int J Recent Trends Sci Technol. 2013;9(2):176–7.

8. Jona JZ, Belin RP. Intramural tracheoesophageal fistula (TEF) associated with esophageal web. J Pediatr Surg. 1977;12(2):227–32. https://doi.org/10.1016/S0022-3468(77)80012-2.

9. Margarit J, Castanon M, Ribo JM, Rodo J, Muntaner A, Lee KW, et al. Congenital esophageal stenosis associated with tracheoesophageal fistula. Pediatr Surg Int. 1994;9:577–8. https://doi.org/10.1007/BF00179686.

10. Gilat T, Rozen P. Fiberoptic endoscopic diagnosis and treatment of a congenital esophageal diaphragm. Am J Dig Dis. 1975;20(8):781–5. https://doi.org/10.1007/BF01070837.

11. Chao H-C, Chen S-Y, Kong M-S. Successful treatment of congenital esophageal web by endoscopic electrocauterlzaion and balloon dilatation. J Pediatr Surg. 2008;43:e13–5. https://doi.org/10.1016/j.jpedsurg.2007.08.059.

12. Patel PC, Yates JA, Gibson WS, Wood WE. Congenital esophageal webs. Int J Pediatr Otorhinolaryngol. 1997;42(2):141–7. https://doi.org/10.1016/S0165-5876(97)00131-6.

13. Roy GR, Cohen RC, Williams SJ. Endoscopic laser division of an esophageal web in a child. J Pediatr Surg. 1966;31:439–40. https://doi.org/10.1016/S0022-3468(96)90757-5.

Chapter 11
Congenital Esophageal Stenosis in Adults

There are few reports about congenital esophageal stenosis in adults. It is thought that it is a rare disease confined to infancy and childhood. McNally et al. in 1993 [1] reported a case of a 31-year-old female with CES who presented with symptoms of non-cardiac esophageal chest pain due to esophageal dysmotility. The patient was diagnosed by EUS as a FMD subtype of CES. The case was treated by esophageal dilatation. Younes et al. reported ten patients with meat impaction and dysphagia due to trachea-like multiple submucosal rings as seen by endoscopy in the mid esophagus. The age ranged from 11 to 75 years with a mean of 27 years. Only one patient had distal reflux esophagitis. Esophageal balloon dilatation in nine patients and Savary dilators in one patient were successful without complications. The authors concluded that CES is an under-recognized cause for long standing dysphagia in adults [2]. Katzka et al. in 2000 [3], reported five cases of CES in only 2 years between the ages of 19 and 46 years. All patients were wrongly diagnosed as reflux strictures, webs or idiopathic pathology. All patients had chronic dysphagia to solids. The stenosis was in the proximal esophagus in 4 and throughout the esophagus in one. Radiographic and endoscopic examination showed smooth concentric stricture or multiple rings similar to tracheal rings. Two patients had EUS which showed focal circumferential hypoechoic wall thickening with disruption of the normal layer pattern corresponding to the areas of luminal narrowing. All patients responded well to dilatation. The authors concluded that CES is a more common condition than previously recognized and that many cases have been misdiagnosed. They hypothesized that this lesion is congenital because of its characteristics, which are similar to those described in infants and children. The main line of treatment is vigorous dilatation accepting the accompanied chest pain. Endoscopic ultrasound is important to confirm the diagnosis.

Oh et al. in 2001 [4], reported seven cases of CES in adults whom double-contrast esophagogram revealed characteristic findings with multiple ring like constrictions in the region of the stricture. Pathologic specimens for histologic examination were not obtained since patients responded to dilatations. However the diagnosis of CES

© Springer Nature Switzerland AG 2019
A. Ibrahim, T. Al-Malki, *Congenital Esophageal Stenosis*,
https://doi.org/10.1007/978-3-030-10782-6_11

depended on the following criteria: (1) Long history of dysphagia for more than 2 years. (2) The presence of strictures diagnosed by esophagogram. (3) No previous history of mediastinal irradiation, caustic ingestion, and drug induced esophagitis, bullous skin diseases. (4) The esophageal mucosa was normal by endoscopy and biopsy. (5) Two patients had endoscopic ultrasonography confirming CES. Clinically, all patients were men having an average age of 38.7 years (range, 19–50 years). All had a long standing history of intermittent, non-progressive dysphagia to solid food. The average duration of symptoms was 8 years (range, 2–17 years). Radiologically, double contrast esophagogram revealed smooth tapered strictures in all seven patients. The stricture was located in the upper esophagus in three patients, the middle third in three and in the lower third in one patient. The average length of the stricture was 4.6 cm (range, 2–7 cm). The average narrowest width was 1.4 cm (range, 0.6–2.5 cm). In all cases, the strictures contained smooth straight ring like constrictions. The average number of constrictions was 5.6 (range, 4–9 constrictions). The distance between constrictions was 1–2 mm in six patients and 1 cm in one patient [4]. There was also mild GER in one patient, a small hiatal hernia in another, and abnormal esophageal motility in another with weakened amplitude of peristalsis and non-peristaltic contractions. Endoscopically, strictures with cartilage like rings with normal overlying mucosa were confirmed in all six patients examined. In one patient biopsy specimen near the GIJ was suggestive of Barrett's esophagus. Endoscopic ultrasonography in the two patients showed circumferential, hypoechoic wall thickening of the esophagus in the stenotic area with disruption of the normal wall layers at this level. This important study gave us important lessons on the topic of CES in general and specifically in adults. Patients with severe forms typically will present early in the neonatal period or early in infancy [5]. Patients with mild forms of CES may present later in older children or even in adults with long standing non progressive dysphagia or food impaction. CES in adults is more common in men and more commonly than is usually recognized. Careful history taking may reveal recognized symptoms early in childhood. We reported a case of CES discovered early in infancy. The patient was dilated once then disappeared for 4 years and came in the OPD with hugely dilated esophagus with only mild symptoms and required another session of dilatation (Fig. 11.1a, b). A double contrast esophagogram can easily diagnose cartilaginous ring-like constrictions that can be missed on a single-contrast barium studies. Despite of the absence of a histological diagnosis yet the diagnosis of cartilaginous origin could be made by endoscopy and endoscopic ultrasonography. These cartilaginous rings can affect the upper, middle or lower esophagus. TBR are said to be refractory to dilatations and frequently require resection. In adults TBR may respond to dilatations. Even in neonates, we reported a case with TBR diagnosed by histology at the anastomotic site responded nicely to a single dilatation [5]. So, dilatation should always be the initial step in managing CES even if it is suspected to be TBR. Careful long term follow up of cases with CES is essential. Recurrence of symptoms is frequent and further sessions of dilatations may be required. Tabira et al. [6] reported a case of squamous cell carcinoma arising on CES in a 65-year-old

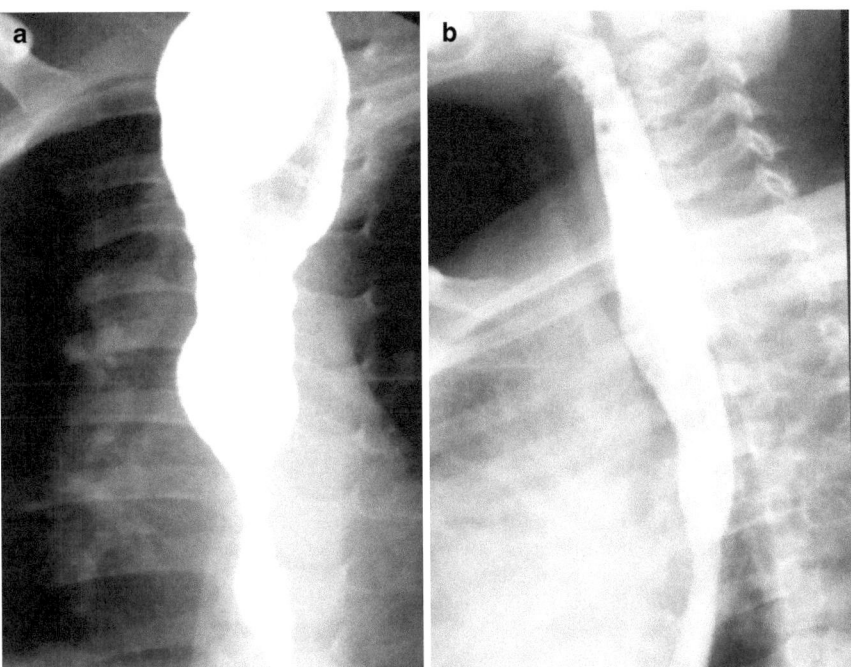

Fig. 11.1 A known case of CES diagnosed in the early infancy, treated by one session of balloon dilatation and the patient disappeared for 4 years. (**a**) hugely dilated esophagus with minimal symptoms at second presentation after 3 years (probably tracheal rings in the esophagus which have never been reported at that age before). (**b**) after successful dilatation

man. The patient had mid symptoms of dysphagia and vomiting since birth and had received no treatment up to age of 20 years when dysphagia became severe requiring several sessions of balloon dilatation with only transient improvement. Transhiatal esophagectomy was performed and the histological examination showed a squamous cell carcinoma on top of FMD.

Gonzalez et al. [7], reported a 27-year-old male, a known case of CES under esophageal dilatation who sustained an esophageal perforation during a dilatation procedure which was treated conservatively. Two years later he presented with spontaneous esophageal perforation proved by CT and oral contrast which revealed a tear in the mid-esophagus with air and contrast in the mediastinum adjacent to the esophagus. A 7-mm tear was identified intraoperatively in the right mid-esophagus which was repaired. However dysphagia is the main presenting feature in adults and older children. Rastogi et al. in 2016 [8], reported an 11-year old boy with dysphagia due to an esophageal web treated with endoscopic dilatation and resection of the web. Interestingly, this patient did not have any history of dysphagia, choking or respiratory symptoms before 2 years when he started to complain. This signifies the fact that minor degrees of stenosis is often overlooked.

References

1. McNally PR, Lemon JC, Goff JS, Freeman SR. Congenital esophageal stenosis presenting as noncardiac, esophageal chest pain. Dig Dis Sci. 1993;38(2):369–73. https://doi.org/10.1007/BF01307558.
2. Younes Z, Johnson DA. Congenital esophageal stenosis: clinical and endoscopic features in adults. Dig Dis. 1999;17:172–7. https://doi.org/10.1159/000016922.
3. Katzka DA, Levine MS, Ginsberg GG, Hammod R, Katz PO, Insko EK, et al. Congenital stenosis in adults. Am J Gastroenterol. 2000;95:32–6. https://doi.org/10.1111/j.1572-0241.2000.01668.x.
4. Oh CH, Levine MS, Katazka DA, Rubesin SE, Pinheiro LW, Igor L. Congenital esophageal stenosis in adults: clinical and radiographic findings in seven patients. AJR. 2001;176:1179–82. https://doi.org/10.2214/ajr.176.5.1761179.
5. Ibrahim AHM, Bazeed MF, Jamil S, Hamad HA, Abdel Raheem IM, Ashraf I. Management of congenital esophageal stenosis associated with esophageal atresia and its impact on postoperative esophageal stricture. Ann Pediatr Surg. 2016;12:36–4. https://doi.org/10.1097/01.XPS.0000482656.06000.84.
6. Tabira Y, Yasunaga M, Sakaguchi T, Okuma T, Yamaguchi Y, Kuhara H, et al. Adult case of squamous cell carcinoma arising on congenital esophageal stenosis due to fibromuscular hypertrophy. Dis Esophagus. 2002;15(4):336–9. https://doi.org/10.1046/j.1442-2050.2002.00270.x.
7. Gonzalez A, Craft CM, Knight TT, Messerschmidt WH. Superimposed spontaneous esophageal perforation in congenital esophageal stenosis. Ann Thorac Surg. 2004;77:1098–100. https://doi.org/10.1016/S0003-4975(03)00890-7.
8. Rastogi R, Majid A, Singh VP, Joon P, Gupta Y. Congenital esophageal stenosis: a rare case of childhood dysphagia. J Gastrointest Dig Syst. 2016;6:1–3. https://doi.org/10.4172/2161-069X.1000407.

Chapter 12
Future Directions for CES

The problems of esophageal motility disorder after successful repair of EA or in cases of isolated CES warrants further investigations. Gross histopathologic, point-count morphometric studies, together with ultrastructural, histochemical, Immunohistochemical studies are required to identify the etiology of motility disorders in CES with or without EA. The results can be correlated with the follow up of the clinical picture of the patients together with radiological and manometric studies of esophageal motility disorders. Sophisticated tests like endoscopic sonography (EUS), high resolution manometry (HRM), pressure flow analysis (PFA), and impedance PFA might be possible in infants and young children. In this aspect, we expect the use of EUS to play a wider diagnostic role for CES and its subtypes in the future. Large series of patients are required from multi centers to reach to a unified consensus for managing cases of CES.

Emerging procedures like peroral endoscopic myotomy (POEM) and esophageal stenting are encouraging to be used in children and probably in infants as well.

The POEM for Children

The peroral endoscopic myotomy (POEM) is a new transesophageal endoscopic approach for treatment of cardiac achalasia which is extremely rare in children. There is no etiological therapies that can restore the normal esophageal peristalsis and function of the lower esophageal sphincter. The present modalities of treatments aim at relieving dysphagia and other symptoms. The available methods of treatments in children are esophageal balloon dilatation and Heller's myotomy. The benefits of balloon dilatation seem to vanish with time and recurrences in children with cardiac achalasia are likely to be more frequent in young age [1, 2]. Laparoscopic Heller's myotomy loses the tactile discrimination between CES

© Springer Nature Switzerland AG 2019
A. Ibrahim, T. Al-Malki, *Congenital Esophageal Stenosis*,
https://doi.org/10.1007/978-3-030-10782-6_12

and achalasia cardia in infants and young children if this differentiation is not possible preoperatively. The POEM procedure was first introduced in children in a 3-year old girl with severe growth retardation, achalasia, and Down syndrome by Maselli in 2012 [3]. The procedure is minimally invasive, less traumatic, less expensive than a surgical procedure, relatively easy in expert hands, and associated with an extremely fast recovery with low complication rate and excellent short term results [1, 4]. However, preoperative differentiation between CES and achalasia is essential if there are hopes that this procedure can be performed for CES in children in the future. POEM is not associated with an antireflux procedure. During POEM, the entire natural anti reflux mechanisms are not touched. The true incidence of GERD after POEM is not known and can be treated conservatively. If the incidence of symptomatic GERD after POEM should be significant, this could impair the acceptance of the procedure.

Nabi et al. [4] reported 15 children who underwent POEM on diagnosed cardiac achalasia using the standard diagnostic modalities like timed barium esophagogram, high resolution manometry and upper GI endoscopy. This is essential to avoid confusion with CES which may not respond d to myotomy (especially the TBR subtype). These authors also mentioned that young patients do not respond well to balloon dilatations and that laparoscopic Heller's myotomy appear to have a more durable relief of symptoms. However, post-operative intervention (including balloon dilation and redo myotomy) was required in 28%of cases on follow up [5]. Another study showed almost the same post-operative results [6]. Nabi et al. [4] reported that they found POEM to be very safe and effective in the pediatric age group, with no major adverse effects. They also mentioned that the response to POEM was durable in their study as evident by persistent symptoms relief and objective parameters like timed barium esophagogram. None of the children required second operation like balloon dilatations or laparoscopic Heller's myotomy. They also mentioned that at present, the role of POEM is not established in pediatric patients with achalasia. They believe that excellent short term results warrants further evaluation of this novel technique in larger trials.

Kethman et al. [7] reported a prospective case series of 10 children with manometry-confirmed achalasia who underwent POEM procedures. The age ranged from 7 to 17 years (mean = 13.4). Their conclusion was that the POEM procedure can be successfully completed in children for the treatment of achalasia. Results demonstrated short-term post-operative improvement in symptoms. The adoption of advanced endoscopic techniques by pediatric surgeons may enable the development of unique intraluminal approaches to congenital anomalies and other childhood diseases [7].

The possibility of using this procedure in CES especially FMD subtypes that fail to improve with balloon dilatation may be great. We hope that trials may include cases of CES in the future.

Esophageal Stents for Children

A removable covered esophageal stent allowed its use in children and expanded the indications for its usage to include a wide variety of congenital and acquired esophageal strictures. Despite the fact that there is no specially designed stents in children, stents have gained acceptance in pediatrics for treatment of recurrent and refractory strictures when medical and endoscopic treatments fail [8]. Esophageal stents became popular in the last decade for the treatment of benign esophageal stricture. Stenting is a new strategy to avoid multiple dilatations in cases of refractory and recurrent stricture. It is less invasive than repeated dilatations and heroic surgeries to replace the esophagus. Stents avoid repeated anesthesia, improves motility, prevent recurrence and are well tolerated.

There are 4 main types of stents in common use: self-expandable metal stent (SEMs), self-expandable plastic stents (SEPSs), biodegradable stents (BDSs), and the custom dynamic stent. A custom dynamic stent fashioned from nasogastric tubes and covered with silicon drainage tubing was successfully used [9]. Contrary to other stents where food passes within the stent, the food in the dynamic stent passes between the stent and the esophageal wall allowing long term improvement of esophageal patency. The dynamic stents improve esophageal motility unlike the widespread self-expandable plastic or metallic esophageal stents [9, 10].

In the future, novel fully covered (biodegradable) stents will be developed with optimal characteristics for refractory benign esophageal stricture (RBES) management. Stents will have a sufficiently high radial force and elasticity to reduce the risk of stent migration and tissue ingrowth, but also a low axial force, reducing severe adverse events and fistula formation. Furthermore, a combination of currently available modalities can be used together such as endoscopic electrocautery incisions and esophageal stenting [11]. A typical example is the novel technique study performed by Liu et al. [12], when the authors used endoscopic incision with esophageal stent placement for the treatment of refractory benign esophageal strictures. Plastic and metallic self-expanding stents were effective in all patients with esophageal perforations [13]. They are very effective for treating post-dilatation perforations and post-anastomotic leaks. Stents are not devoid of complications in pediatric patients. Gagging, stent displacement and migration into the stomach have been reported. Life threatening events such as perforation, air way compression, granulation tissue formation, and GERD or aspiration pneumonia are also reported. The most significant complication is stent erosion causing arterioesophageal fistula with the danger of massive bleeding and even mortality [11, 14].

Esophageal stenting is a promising tool for the treatment of recurrent and refractory esophageal strictures. They have the advantage of maintaining luminal patency for long periods as well as better oral feeding. However, there are problems of patient intolerance to the stent and other complications mentioned above. Prospective trials are required to demonstrate long-term efficacy and safety. Better quality stents, improvement in the techniques and protocols for stenting hold hopes for better results without complications in the future.

References

1. Familiari P, Marchese M, Giganti G, Boskoski I, Tringali A, Perri V, et al. Peroral endoscopic myotomy for the treatment of achalasia in children. J Pediatr Gastroenterol Nutr. 2013;57:794–7. https://doi.org/10.1097/MPG.0b013e3182a803f7.
2. Hulselmans M, Vanuytsel T, Degreef T, Sifrim D, Coosemans W, Lerut T, et al. Long-term outcome of pneumatic dilatation in the treatment of achalasia. Clin Gastroenterol Hepatol. 2010;8:30–5. https://doi.org/10.1016/j.cgh.2009.09.020.
3. Maselli R, Inoue H, Misawa M, Ikeda H, Hosoya T, Onimaru M, et al. Peroral endoscopic myotomy (POEM) in a 3-year old girl with severe growth retardation, achalasia, and Down syndrome. Endoscopy. 2012;44:E285–7. https://doi.org/10.1055/s-0032-1309924.
4. Nabi Z, Ramchandani M, Reddy DN, Darisetty S, Kotla R, Kalapala R, et al. Per oral endoscopic myotomy in children with achalasia cardia. J Neurogastroenterol Motil. 2016;22(4):613–9. https://doi.org/10.5056/jnm15172.
5. Pachl MJ, Rex D, Decoppi P, Cross K, Kiely EM, Drake D, et al. Paediatric laparoscopic Heller's cardiomyotomy: a single center series. J Pediatr Surg. 2014;49:289–92. https://doi.org/10.1016/j.jpedsurg.2013.11.042.
6. Askegard-Giesmann JR, Grams JM, Hanna AM, Iqbal CW, Teh S, Moir CR. Minimally invasive Heller's myotomy in children: safe and effective. J Pediatr Surg. 2009;44:909–11. https://doi.org/10.1016/j.jpedsurg.2009.01.022.
7. Kethman WC, Thoson CM, Sinclair TJ, Berquist WE, Chao SD, Wall JK. Initial experience with peroral endoscopic myotomy for treatment of achalasia in children. J Pediatr Surg. 2018;53:1532. https://doi.org/10.1016/j.jpedsurg.2017.07.023.
8. Dall'Oglio L, Caldaro T, Foschia F, Faraci S, Federrici di Abriola G, Rea F, et al. Endoscopic management of esophageal stenosis in children: new and traditional treatments. World J Gastrointest Endosc. 2016;8(4):212–9. https://doi.org/10.4253/wjge.v8.i4.212.
9. Foschia F, De Angelis P, Torroni F, Romeo E, Caldaro T, di Abriola GF, Pane A, et al. Custom dynamic stent for esophageal strictures in children. J Pediatric Surg. 2011;46(5):848–53. https://doi.org/10.1016/j.jpedsurg.2011.02.014.
10. Caldaro T, Torroni F, De Angelis P, Foschia F, Rea F, Romeo E, et al. Dynamic esophageal stents. Dis Esophagus. 2013;26:388–91. https://doi.org/10.1111/dote.12048.
11. Siersema PD. Treatment of refractory being esophageal strictures: it is all about being "patient". Gastrointest Endosc. 2016;84(2):229–31. https://doi.org/10.1016/j.gie.2016.04.035.
12. Liu D, Tan Y, Wang Y, Zhang J, Zhou J, Duan T, et al. Endoscopic incision with esophageal stent placement for the treatment of benign esophageal strictures. Gastrointest Endosc. 2015;81:1036–40. https://doi.org/10.1016/j.gie.2014.10.037.
13. Manfredi MA, Jennings RW, Anjum MW, Hamilton TE, Smithers CJ, Lightdale JR. Externally removable stents in the treatment of benign recalcitrant strictures and esophageal perforations in pediatric patients with esophageal atresia. Gastrointest Endosc. 2014;80:246–52. https://doi.org/10.1016/j.gie.2014.01.033.
14. Baird R, Laberge JM, Lévesque D. Anastomotic stricture after esophageal atresia repair: a critical review of recent literature. Eur J Pediatr Surg. 2013;23:204–13. https://doi.org/10.1055/s-0033-1347917.

Summary and Conclusions

- CES is rare but common if associated with EA.
- The etiology of esophageal dysfunction in CES is complex. It can be due to CES itself or associated EA or both in combination. It includes textural abnormalities, excessive dissection, GER and the development of stricture. The muscles may be hypoplastic, Hypertrophic, distorted by fibrosis, cartilage and/or respiratory glands. There are abnormalities in the intrinsic and extrinsic innervation of both esophageal pouches. Neuropeptides are also abnormal. Lack of nitric oxide (NO) inhibitory innervation may be an important mechanism in the pathogenesis of stenosis and dysmotility. Also, there are ultrastructural abnormalities in EA.
- The present definition of CES proposed by Fékété is excellent for the intrinsic intramural part of the disease. The definition needs to be revised to include the spectrum of CES.
- CES can affect the anastomotic site of EA, extends distally to the cardia or be a separate distal CES away from the anastomosis and cardia.
- IF the CES involves the GEJ, it behaves like achalasia cardia with diagnostic challenges.
- CES is a spectrum of diseases that can behave differently according to the type, site and severity.
- The true incidence of CES is not known due to difficulties in diagnosis, successful dilatation and failure to obtain a histological diagnosis.
- There are difficulties in diagnosing CES in neonates due to absence of histology specimens and lack of a high index of suspicion during initial esophagogram after primary repair.
- Lack of miniprobe endoscopic ultrasonography (MEUS) facility and expertise adds to the diagnostic difficulties of CES.
- The presentation of CES can be acute and stormy in the neonatal period or it can be delayed most commonly to the weaning period. The course of the disease can be benign to present in late infancy, childhood or even in adults.
- CES can be a risk factor for anastomotic leak, recurrent TEF, refractory and recurrent esophageal stricture.

© Springer Nature Switzerland AG 2019
A. Ibrahim, T. Al-Malki, *Congenital Esophageal Stenosis*,
https://doi.org/10.1007/978-3-030-10782-6

- Neonatal diagnosis of CES can be improved by a routine passage of a transanastomotic size 8 NGT during primary repair, obtaining biopsies from the tips of esophageal pouches for histology and having a high index of suspicion during initial esophagogram. Anastomotic leak or recurrent TEF can be a shadow for a distal CES.
- Intolerance to feeds, recurrent respiratory symptoms (apnea, desaturations, aspiration, and choking…) are the main symptoms in neonates and young infants. Foreign body impaction and dysphagia are the main symptoms in older children.
- The triad of stenosis, dysmotility and GER is not uncommon in CES associated with EA sparing the GEJ.
- Successful NGT feeding is a good test to diagnose obstruction at the esophageal level.
- Esophagogram (with a low threshold for repetition), PH, impedance studies, upper endoscopy, esophageal manometry, and EUS are important tools to differentiate CES from cardiac achalasia and reflux esophagitis.
- Intra operative palpation for CES and/or frozen section biopsies are helpful in doubtful cases of CES if EUS is not available.
- The initial line of treatment is always dilatation whatever the type of CES is. The type of stenosis then determines the modality of treatment as diagnosed by EUS to achieve successful results without undue prolonged courses of dilatations and complications.
- Many cases diagnosed as neonatal or infantile cardiac achalasia are probably cases of CES that either require resection after failure of Heller's myotomy (TBR) or respond to dilatation or myotomy if it is FMD subtype.
- Isolated CES responds better to treatment than CES associated with EA.
- Gastrostomy and partial fundoplication may become mandatory should the triad of stenosis, dysmotility and GER develop.
- No heroic esophageal replacement surgery except after full chance of conservative management has been offered.

Recommendations

- Obtaining histopathologic samples from the tips of the esophageal pouches routinely during primary repair are helpful for early diagnosis of CES in the neonatal period.
- A transanastomotic size 8 Fr NGT is mandatory to rule out CES during primary.
- A high index of suspicion should be practiced during the initial esophagogram. Consider anastomotic leak and recurrent TEF as a possible shadow for a distal CES.
- A low threshold for repeating esophagogram is required if still in doubt.
- Early diagnosis and prophylactic dilatation should start as early as 4 weeks after primary repair of EA.
- The miniprobe EUS is helpful for the diagnosis of CES and its subtypes and the decision about the treatment modality and should be used in a wider scale.
- Protracted courses of dilatations with adjuncts, indwelling balloon dilatations, incisional therapy, and stents are preferable to esophageal replacement surgery despite of the possible complications which we hope to be minimized in the future with better techniques and better quality of stents.

© Springer Nature Switzerland AG 2019

A. Ibrahim, T. Al-Malki, *Congenital Esophageal Stenosis*,

https://doi.org/10.1007/978-3-030-10782-6